Infertility

Infertility

WHAT CAUSES IT AND HOW IT IS TESTED

WHERE TO GO FOR HELP

FERTILITY DRUGS, TREATMENTS AND OPERATIONS

HOW TO COPE IF ALL ELSE FAILS

Roger Neuberg
F. R. C. O. G.

Consultant Obstetrician & Gynaecologist
Director of Infertility Services
Leicester Royal Infirmary
Leicester, U. K.

Thorsons
An Imprint of HarperCollinsPublishers

Thorsons
An Imprint of HarperCollins*Publishers*
77–85 Fulham Palace Road,
Hammersmith, London W6 8JB

Published by Thorsons 1991
10 9 8 7 6 5 4 3

British Library Cataloguing in Publication Data
Neuberg, Roger
  Infertility.
  1. Man. Infertility
  I. Title
  616.692

  ISBN 0-7225-1517-0

Printed and bound in Great Britain by
Caledonian International Book Manufacturing Ltd, Glasgow

And a woman who held a babe against her bosom said, Speak to us of Children.

And he said:

Your children are not your children.

They are the sons and daughters of Life's longing for itself.

They come through you but not from you.

And though they are with you yet they belong not to you.

You may give them your love but not your thoughts.

For they have their own thoughts.

You may house their bodies but not their souls,

For their souls dwell in the house of to-morrow, which you cannot visit, not even in your dreams.

You may strive to be like them, but seek not to make them like you.

For life goes not backward nor tarries with yesterday.

You are the bows from which your children as living arrows are sent forth.

The Archer sees the mark upon the path of the infinite, and He bends you with His might that His arrows may go swift and far.

Let your bending in the Archer's hand be for gladness;

For even as He loves the arrow that flies, so He loves also the bow that is stable.

The Prophet, Kahlil Gibran

Contents

Acknowledgements 11
Foreword 13
Preface 15
Introduction 17

1 How 'normal' fertility works 21

2 Could one of us be infertile? 32

3 The first steps towards finding out 35

4 The Infertility Clinic 46

5 Special investigations 59

6 Should I be on a fertility drug? 79

7 Will an operation help? 107

8 What can be done for the infertile man? 126

9 Assisted conception techniques and other options 138

10 So near and yet so far 172

11 Twenty questions 183

12 Looking to the future 203

13 Coming to terms with childlessness 206

Useful addresses 209
Glossary of terms 213
Index 223

Acknowledgements

I am indebted to my wife Ruth for listening to and for proof-reading every chapter as it was completed. This, added to her own contact with my patients over the years, must mean that by now she knows more about the management of infertility than many doctors! I owe her and the rest of my family my grateful thanks for their understanding, when I disappeared, yet again, to be closeted with my word processor.

I experienced the qualms that every author must have upon handing over his or her creation to a total stranger to edit. What would she do to my 'baby'? My fears were groundless. Sally Crawford of Thorsons turned a phrase here, corrected spelling mistakes and grammatical errors there, and the 'delivery' was without complication. We spent many hours on the telephone discussing different word usages and I must say that I got a great insight into the editor's skills which Sally certainly personifies.

I am most grateful to Parul Patel, illustrator to the Department of Medical Illustration at the Leicester Royal Infirmary, for her faithful redrawing of my own line drawings and diagrams, to make them look the work of a professional.

Finally, and most importantly, to all my infertility patients over the years, I owe an incalculable debt for allowing me the privilege to become part of both their successes and their failures.

Foreword

From any profession 'expert' views are easy to obtain and will often be characterized by their diversity, each expert holding an opinion at variance in some way with that of his or her colleague.

The field of infertility is no exception and it was therefore with some apprehension that I agreed to read and then comment on this book.

Many patients approach BPAS for help with infertility having themselves read books on their perceived problem and thus gaining a range of opinion and probably conflicting advice.

I can now say that, if this book had been the first on a patient's reading list, a great deal of confusion and the anxiety this creates could have been avoided.

Roger Neuberg writes in a simple and understandable way and takes the reader on a clear, guided tour of infertility, its causes and possible solutions.

He does not use his expertise to define and dissect the subject but rather sets a plausible agenda with which readers can relate and utilize for themselves.

I am pleased to record my apprehension was misplaced!

Ian H. Jones
Director
British Pregnancy Advisory Service

Preface

When I was first approached to write this book, I had already written *So you want to have a baby* which is a patient's guide to infertility investigation and management. It was based upon the many verbal explanations that I have given to my own patients over the years. However, this booklet was only 42 pages long and of necessity rather concise. I therefore leapt at the opportunity of considerably enlarging the concept of the booklet. While it is specifically directed to you, the infertile couple, I hope that it will be of interest to others: workers in the field of infertility, whether doctors or nurses, or counsellors who are involved at the 'front line', having to communicate directly with the patient.

Infertility is a rapidly growing sub-speciality of gynaecology and as such is becoming more and more complex as times goes on. Throughout this book, the medical terms will be carefully explained to you as the text unfolds. I make no apologies for the fairly detailed yet, I hope, easy to understand section on how ovulation works, because it is essential in order to understand the problems that can occur and the different infertility treatments that are available.

There is a full discussion on the range of infertility investigations and treatments that are currently in use, as well as their implications and what they involve for you and your partner. So, if there is a sense of familiarity when you meet these tests for the first time, then to some extent I will have succeeded. I will also be making liberal use of patient examples and case histories and there is also a section on patient questions and answers.

To be infertile is bad enough, but there can be additional problems that are actually caused by the investigations and treatments themselves. Being aware of these may reduce the chances of treatment eventually closing in on you and becoming (as it does for many) the sole purpose of your existence. There are better ways of living.

In talking to you through this book I hope that you will be helped to get your problems into some perspective. The majority of you will succeed in having children in your family by some means or another. Sadly, some of you will remain childless in spite of having 'tried everything'. If you should fall into this minority group I hope that at least you will be able to say that 'It wasn't for the want of trying'.

R.N. Leicester 1990

Introduction

In Western societies five out of six couples have no difficulty with conception. Eighty per cent will achieve a pregnancy within the first year of trying and the remainder within the second year. But one in six of us will be infertile. Everything in our society, however, seems to be geared to the fertile: family planning clinics, contraception advice, maternity services, abortion clinics and the provision of male and female sterilization facilities. In contrast, infertility services are few and far between. However, there is a slowly growing public and political awareness of the predicament of the infertile couple in the community.

Virtually from childhood, our expectations are that we will become parents. Most of us take our fertility for granted. Certainly we hear about those who cannot have children for one reason or another, but that applies to *them* . . . other people, not us! Most couples, unless they use contraception, expect a pregnancy to occur within a short space of time. But as time passes, expectation and hope change to doubt and anxiety. Desperation and, if the problem continues, a sense of bitter isolation follows. For the unfortunate minority who cannot be helped to achieve their goal, resignation and hopefully acceptance will be the outcome.

Infertility will not kill you, but God! how it hurts!

Although it's not really a question of fairness, it is only human nature to want to cry out 'IT ISN'T FAIR!' The situation isn't helped by enquiring in-laws hinting that 'It's about time you two started a family,' or 'You're not getting any younger you know.' You *know* it's time, and yes, you are *very* aware of the years going by, THANK YOU VERY MUCH! If, on top of all this, everyone around you seems to be getting pregnant it just highlights your own sense of inadequacy. It's even more difficult to keep smiling as, persistently, friends and other close members of the family prove their own fertility. I have known couples who have actually gone so far as to avoid contact with pregnant friends because it has proved to be too upsetting. After all, when parents of young children get together, the main topic of conversation is going to be how the children are getting on, their adventures and mischief, the choosing of schools and so on. And when they dare to complain at finding themselves pregnant *again* . . .! I have a vivid mental picture of one delightful patient who ran a restaurant and was incensed to overhear a customer complaining to a companion about being pregnant yet again. As the seemingly disgruntled woman left the premises, G. ran out after her and, in bitter frustration, flung handfuls of gravel from the drive in the direction of the unaware dinner guest!

There can be no doubt that infertility causes considerable emotional tension. It is however debatable just how much of that very tension is in itself a *cause* of infertility. The anxiety state in the infertile is a chronic one which is constantly present and increases as month after month goes by. I personally believe that this is at least one factor in infertility. One explanation for this is that it is well known that stress will cause smooth muscle in the body to contract. Examples of this are the contraction of bladder and bowel smooth muscle leading to their frequent emptying when we are particularly apprehensive. It would be most curious if the smooth muscle of the fallopian tubes behaved any differently under stress, especially where each tube enters the muscle wall of uterus (see diagram on page 23). All gynaecologists have seen evidence of spasm (involuntary contraction) of these tubes when testing for blockage; occasionally considerable pressure has to be applied before the injected dye (needed to show up any blockage) will pass out of the uterus into the tubes. Without the 'stress factor' it becomes difficult to explain the numbers of patients with a significant degree of infertility who become pregnant virtually en route to the Infertility Clinic or shortly afterwards. I have become more and more convinced that the relaxation in tension brought about by the feeling that at last something is going to be done to help them is a real factor. I find that one-fifth of my patients who become pregnant do so while only keeping a temperature chart and without any medication whatsoever. Is it perhaps also significant that they will have left the Infertility Clinic with a much more positive outlook and will be very much more relaxed than when they arrived? To look at yet another aspect of stress, nobody would pretend that adoption can cure infertility. But in the cases of some couples whose infertility is unexplained (i.e. no obvious cause has been found when all the relevant tests have been undertaken), the relaxation brought about by the fulfilment of having a child in their family at last, may remove the chronic stress factor. There are many reported instances of pregnancy after adoption in this group of patients. Is this just pure chance?

Many of you will have experienced the feeling of isolation that your infertility has brought to you. But there is much comfort to be gained when you realize that you are not on your own. I cannot stress enough the benefits there are in joining patient-orientated self-help groups (page 209). The basic unit of these superb organizations is the local regional group which has the back-up of the main central counselling facilities, excellent fact-sheets and regular up-to-date bulletins. Locally run meetings are informative as well as being fun to attend. Not only are such organizations a source of friends but they will help restore your sense of belonging to a community, instead of the sense of isolation you may be feeling. The articles written in such bulletins are frequently written by infertility experts and I for one am constantly learning from them. Readers' letters help other members to cope with their own problems, especially when they read about other couples who have gone through similar experiences and eventually succeeded in having a baby. Many have been set up for you by infertile couples themselves.

I wholeheartedly recommend them to you.

How 'normal' fertility works

At first it seems as if it must be so simple to get pregnant. After all it's not something that one needs to have any intelligence to do. And it only takes one sperm to fertilize an egg, doesn't it?

But there's so much more to it than that. 'Getting pregnant' is in fact such a complex procedure that it is quite astonishing that anybody manages it at all!

There is of course some essential equipment that is required in order to bring about a pregnancy. Let us take a look at the male and female anatomy and see how they work (Figs. 1-3).

The lower part of the brain contains a region called the **hypothalamus** which controls a pea-sized structure called the **pituitary gland** (Fig. 4). This gland controls the behaviour of many other glands in the body including the ovaries in the female and the testicles in the male. The pituitary gland controls these distant glands by releasing messenger substances called hormones into the bloodstream. The ovary responds by maturing an egg and the testicles by producing sperm. Sperm production is a continuous process and the normally fertile man is fertile every day from puberty until old age. In contrast, the production of a mature egg is a single event that occurs once in each menstrual cycle.

In the ovaries, egg **follicles** also grow continuously and at all ages, from infancy to the menopause ('change of life'). However, most of these follicles only grow to a limited degree and are never released as mature eggs. At birth the ovaries contain over a million egg follicles. Only about 350 are ever ovulated.

At the beginning of a period, the start of a new menstrual cycle, the hypothalamus signals to the pituitary to release a hormone called **Follicle Stimulating Hormone (FSH)**. FSH stimulates a group of about 20 follicles to undergo further growth (Fig. 5).

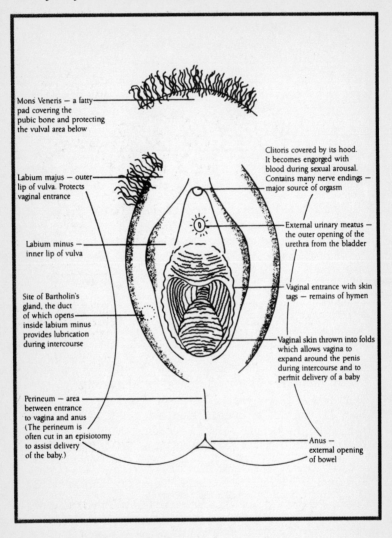

Mons Veneris — a fatty pad covering the pubic bone and protecting the vulval area below

Clitoris covered by its hood. It becomes engorged with blood during sexual arousal. Contains many nerve endings — major source of orgasm

Labium majus — outer lip of vulva. Protects vaginal entrance

External urinary meatus — the outer opening of the urethra from the bladder

Labium minus — inner lip of vulva

Vaginal entrance with skin tags — remains of hymen

Site of Bartholin's gland, the duct of which opens inside labium minus provides lubrication during intercourse

Vaginal skin thrown into folds which allows vagina to expand around the penis during intercourse and to permit delivery of a baby

Perineum — area between entrance to vagina and anus (The perineum is often cut in an episiotomy to assist delivery of the baby.)

Anus — external opening of bowel

Fig. 1: Female anatomy (external).

During the next two weeks, as these follicles develop, they produce an increasing quantity of a female hormone called **oestrogen**. The oestrogen enters the bloodstream and feeds back to the pituitary gland where it is recognized by special receptors. This 'feedback' leads to a reduction in FSH output (Fig. 6).

The reduction in available FSH means that there is only sufficient

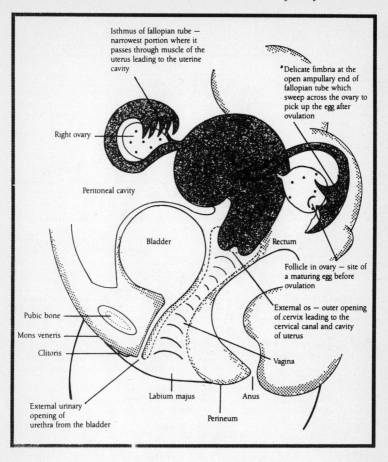

Isthmus of fallopian tube —
narrowest portion where it
passes through muscle of the
uterus leading to the uterine
cavity

*Delicate fimbria at the
open ampullary end of
fallopian tube which
sweep across the ovary to
pick up the egg after
ovulation

Right ovary

Peritoneal cavity

Bladder

Rectum

Follicle in ovary — site of
a maturing egg before
ovulation

External os — outer opening
of cervix leading to the
cervical canal and cavity
of uterus

Pubic bone

Mons veneris

Clitoris

Vagina

External urinary
opening of
urethra from the bladder

Labium majus

Anus

Perineum

Fig. 2: Female anatomy (internal).

for the most advanced follicle in the group of 20 to be able to continue
to develop to full maturity. The others shrink. This explains why
pregnancy in the human usually only results in a single baby.

The rapidly rising oestrogen from the single maturing follicle now
triggers off the release of another hormone from the pituitary called
Luteinizing Hormone (LH). About 28-32 hours after the surge in LH
production, the mature egg is released from the follicle. This is called
ovulation (Fig. 7).

After ovulation the empty follicle forms a structure called the
corpus luteum which produces the second female hormone called

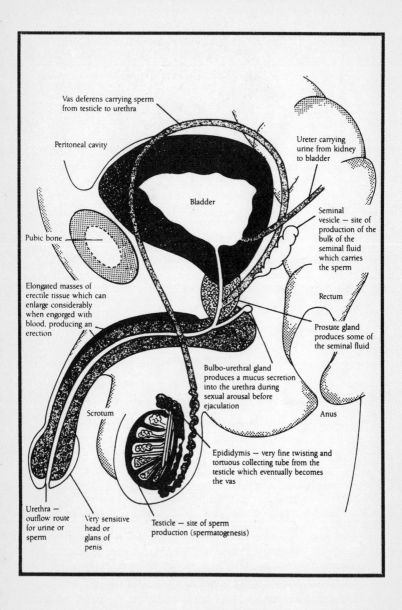

Fig. 3: Male anatomy (internal).

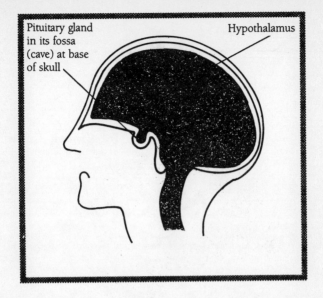

Fig. 4: The centres in the brain that control hormone release.

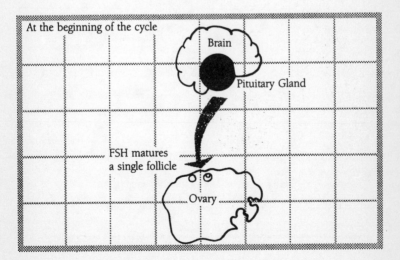

Fig. 5: The hormone pathway that stimulates the ovary to bring egg-containing follicles to maturation.

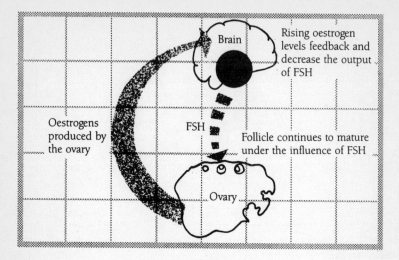

Fig. 6: The hormone pathway that stimulates the ovary to mature an egg.

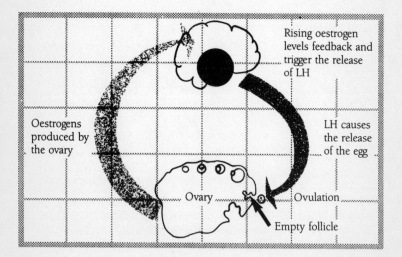

Fig. 7: The hormone pathway that stimulates the ovary to release an egg.

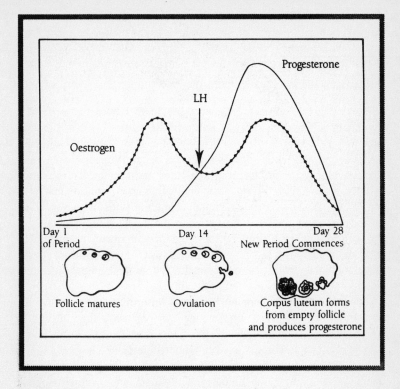

Fig. 8: Changes in the outputs of oestrogen and progesterone by the ovary throughout the menstrual cycle.

progesterone. The level of progesterone rises after ovulation and, with an additional production of oestrogen, brings the lining (**endometrium**) of the uterus into a state of readiness to receive a fertilized egg. If a fertilized egg does not implant, the progesterone level slowly falls and a period commences. The whole cycle now begins once more (Fig. 8).

The acidity of the vagina is in fact very hostile to sperm, so that any sperm that are left in the vagina are rapidly destroyed. This may not seem to be the best way of helping reproduction but vaginal acidity is important as a protective against certain infections. The sperm are, however, given temporary protection by the alkalinity of the semen which allows sufficient time (seconds as opposed to minutes) for the sperm to 'escape' into the haven of the alkaline mucus of the cervix (neck of the womb).

Of the 200-300 million sperm that will be ejaculated into the vagina at intercourse, the vast majority are lost, either destroyed by vaginal acidity or escaping with seminal fluid that trickles out of the vagina. Yet other sperm may be engulfed by cells of the endometrium (the lining of the uterus) or pass along the fallopian tubes to be lost within the peritoneal cavity of the abdomen.

The cervical mucus is only favourable to sperm for a few days before ovulation occurs. During this 'fertile phase' of the cycle the mucus becomes very stretchable and flowing. Microscopic open 'pathways' in the mucus guide the sperm into crypts or reservoirs in the cervical canal where they can be stored safely and then released at intervals into the cavity of the uterus. This means that an egg may be fertilized even if intercourse does not exactly coincide with ovulation. This temporary and often very short storage of the sperm provides a short incubation period during which time they acquire the ability to fertilize an egg, a process called **capacitation**. (Any abnormal sperm are not able to reach the safety of the crypts in the cervix quickly enough and are destroyed.)

Involuntary contractions of the uterus rapidly move the sperm up into the fallopian tubes which they can reach within minutes of insemination. But the degree of sperm loss is so great that only a tiny minority, a few hundred, actually reach the egg.

After ovulation, the egg, with its surrounding follicle cells, sticks for a while to the surface of the ovary. The muscular movements of the fallopian tube enable the fimbrial end to move across the surface of the ovary and pick up the egg. It is here within the ampullary (flask-like) end of the tube that fertilization occurs.

The egg remains fertilizable for up to 24 hours. The fertilizable life of sperm is up to 48 hours. It is now known that in a natural cycle most women will ovulate during the late afternoon. So there is some advantage in having intercourse in the morning of the day of ovulation. This will give the sperm sufficient time to reach the end of the tube and act as a reception committee for the arrival of the egg! The egg does not appear to attract sperm to it. It seems to be pure chance whether or not the sperm make contact with the egg in the ampulla of the tube (Fig. 9).

Around the egg is a layer called the **zona pellucida** which only permits a single sperm to penetrate it, and then forms an impenetrable barrier to all other sperm. The head of the fertilizing sperm then releases its contents which move towards the nucleus of the egg. The egg has now been fertilized. The first cell division then

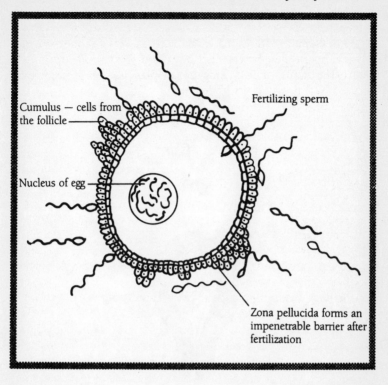

Cumulus — cells from the follicle

Fertilizing sperm

Nucleus of egg

Zona pellucida forms an impenetrable barrier after fertilization

Fig. 9: Sperm swim around the egg until one is able to penetrate and fertilize it.

takes place, first into 2 cells then 4, 8, 16, etc. The muscular action of the fallopian tube and the current of movement set up by the cilia (fine hairs on some of the cells lining the intricate canal of the tube) transports the new **embryo** towards the uterus. It takes about 30 hours for the embryo, now called a **morula**, to reach the **isthmus** (narrowing) of the tube where it remains for another 30 hours before entering the uterus. If the tube has become distorted by previous infection or surgery, the embryo can get stuck within the tube, a potentially dangerous condition that gives rise to an **ectopic** pregnancy.

Once the embryo reaches the uterus it takes another three days before **implantation** occurs. A space appears in the morula (now known as a **blastocyst**) and the blastocyst makes contact with and actually invades the endometrium to become engulfed by it. The pregnancy therefore grows within the wall of the uterus and bulges into the uterine cavity as it enlarges (Fig. 10).

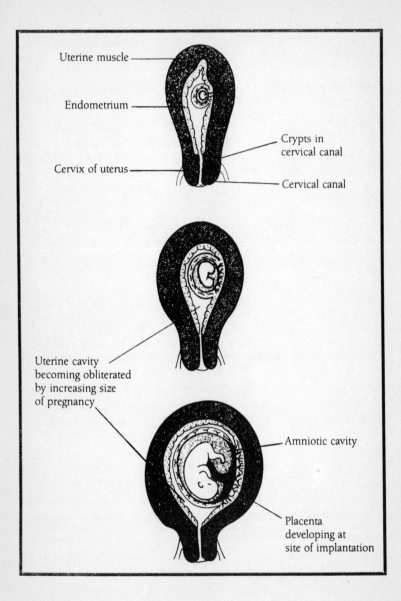

Fig. 10: The stages from implantation of the embryo to formation and growth of the fetus.

It is during this time of implantation that the pregnancy first produces a hormone called **Human Chorionic Gonadotrophin (HCG)**. All pregnancy tests are based upon the detection of this hormone.

To sum up, in order for a pregnancy to occur, the following stages are necessary:

- Ovulation is vital.
- Intercourse must take place during the fertile phase.
- The sperm count must be adequate in order that a sufficient number of sperm may reach the egg.
- The cervical mucus must not be hostile to the sperm.
- There must not be any obstruction to fertilization taking place, such as blocked tubes preventing the sperm from reaching the egg, or adhesions around the ovaries preventing the egg from reaching the tube.

Could one of us be infertile?

Infertility means different things to different people. Here are a few examples:

Hansaben and Ramesh have been married for six months and are becoming alarmed that no pregnancy has occurred when they almost expected it to result from their honeymoon!

Carole and David have taken no contraceptive precautions for three years and are beginning to wonder if all is well.

Janet and Stephen had no difficulty in conceiving their first child and now find that they are not increasing the size of their family in the way that they had hoped.

Are all three couples infertile? And just what do doctors regard as 'infertility' anyway? Well, to answer that let us first take a look at *normal* fertility. In the normal fertile couple there is about a one in three chance of a pregnancy occurring in each cycle of uncontracepted intercourse. As has been mentioned, the vast majority of normally fertile couples will achieve a pregnancy within two years of trying. By this timescale, Hansaben and Ramesh who have only been trying for a family for six months, can hardly be regarded as being infertile. But this doesn't necessarily mean that investigations shouldn't begin this early. For example, if you are only having 1-2 periods a year you will only have 1-2 chances a year of becoming pregnant instead of the normal 12-13. In these circumstances, having to wait for a regulation 'year or two' before seeking help seems a rather pointless delaying exercise. Some women may only have had their first opportunity of becoming pregnant in their late thirties because of a late marriage. If this is the case then time is precious and early investigation would be wise.

Carole and David, who have had several years of uncontracepted intercourse without a pregnancy, may very well have a problem and should seek prompt advice rather than let the years flow past. Sometimes a woman will delay starting a family until her late thirties for a variety of reasons. It may be that she has a very fulfilling career with prospects of promotion. A career is every bit as important to a woman as to a man, but to many women, so too is the additional career of being a mother. While many women have had baby after baby right into their mid-forties, female fertility does tend to reduce gradually from the age of 30 and more rapidly from the age of 35. Sadly, all too often couples only seek professional help in a panic when many years have passed and it is too late to consider some of the options that would be available to them when they were younger. But to go to the other extreme is almost as bad. I have known women who have not taken up the opportunity of promotion because they are 'trying for a family and it wouldn't be fair to my employers if I became pregnant straight away'. But that pregnancy may never happen and the promotion chance may never come again. One should live and enjoy living. A job can always be given up later or maternity leave taken if that is preferred. Worst of all is to give up a fulfilling career in the belief that to do so may help one to become pregnant; it may not.

Janet and Stephen would appear to have what is called secondary infertility. One could argue that they do after all have a child already and shouldn't really be getting too intense over their lack of success in increasing their family size. However, for them it's a problem which is causing distress. Some cases of secondary infertility follow a miscarriage or a termination of an earlier unwanted pregnancy. Infertility after a termination is particularly tragic if it is now the same partner with whom the woman is desperately trying to have a family.

But what about the 44-year-old with five children by the same partner, their ages ranging between 19 and 5 years, who claims to be desperate about not having any more? If such a woman is desperate she certainly has a problem, but by no stretch of the imagination could she be regarded as being truly infertile. Time has simply run out for her.

So when should you do something about what seems to you to be infertility? The answer really is when you feel that you have reason to be worried. The first step is to make an appointment to see your family doctor. The appointment system can be a bit daunting, but not all practice receptionists are dragons trying to protect their treasures (in this case the doctors) from the patients! It is ideal to go together, as a couple, because the problem is after all a joint one. You are also taking along moral support!

It is unlikely that you will get an airy dismissal from your doctor and be told simply to 'get on with it' rather than bother him. The majority of doctors are very well informed about basic infertility problems and are in a position to be able to offer you considerable help and advice. First of all, the caring family doctor can allay unnecessary fears and help you to get your infertility into perspective. Secondly, he can himself organize a number of investigations which may actually pin-point the cause of your infertility. He is also in a position to know about local facilities and where, or to whom, it may be best to refer you.

From the gynaecologists' point of view, it is a delight to receive a referral from a doctor where the couple have already been well 'worked up', that is when most of the basic essential investigations have been carried out, and the results clearly given. It can save you many months of additional delay and frustration. A doctor's referral letter which simply states, 'Dear Dr, Infertility. Please see and advise', will not arouse much interest or enthusiasm at the receiving end! When, eventually, you are due to be seen by a specialist, make sure that you bring any relevant information you may have with you: temperature charts and the results of sperm counts and blood tests are all important. This all helps to avoid delays, and delays are the last thing you will want.

The first steps towards finding out

I have mentioned that there is a great deal that your doctor can do both in assessing your infertility problem and in carrying out some basic investigations. Not only can these tests pin-point the problem that is causing your infertility, but during the months of waiting for your clinic appointment, you can actually be doing something useful. It also means that if the results of basic investigations organized by the doctor are available at the first visit to the Infertility Clinic, hospital treatment can be started promptly without delay.

Rubella antibody screening

Rubella or German Measles is a very mild viral illness that only rarely causes any medical problems; that is, assuming that you are *not* pregnant at the time. If a woman catches Rubella in the first four months of pregnancy, the infection can leave her unborn baby with major handicaps such as deafness, blindness, mental deficiency and heart disease. There can hardly be a worse nightmare than to succeed at long last in getting pregnant, catch Rubella in early pregnancy, and then have to consider whether or not to have that longed-for pregnancy aborted. You *must* make 100 per cent certain that you are immune to Rubella before you even try to become pregnant. It's too uncertain to rely upon your mother telling you that you had German Measles as a child because some childhood virus infections can mimic Rubella. Don't even rely on having had a vaccination as a schoolgirl because 5 per cent of these vaccinations fail to produce immunity. The only way to find out is by means of a very simple blood test that your doctor can send to the nearest Public Health Laboratory. If the test shows that you are not immune then you must be made immune by vaccination. It is very important that the vaccination is given during a normal period when there can be no question of your being pregnant at the time. (The reason for this precaution is that the vaccine is a weakened form of the live virus which if given in pregnancy has a slight chance of damaging the baby.) For the next three months it is essential that contraceptive precautions be taken, again to avoid any chance of the vaccine affecting the baby. I would recommend the use of both the condom (sheath) and a spermidical pessary for contraception. Hormonal contraception such as the Pill or single-dose progesterone injections would certainly stop you ovulating, but could delay the return of your normal cycle. Eight weeks after the vaccination a repeat blood test is taken to measure your antibody response to the vaccination.

Most adults are immune to Rubella whether or not there is any history of ever having had the infection. If you are not immune, however, the investment of only a few weeks of time will not significantly delay your becoming pregnant and could save you untold distress later.

Basal body temperature (BBT) charts

I personally believe that the BBT chart is an extremely useful aid both to the infertile couple and to the Infertility Clinic. It is, however, only useful if you have a reasonably regular menstrual cycle. It is without doubt the simplest, cheapest and least time-consuming method of assessing the apparent normality of ovulation. A number of clinics regard BBT charts as having no place in the modern investigation of infertility and as doing nothing other than to cause additional stress. But anything can be stressful if it is not done correctly. To simply hand you a poor quality BBT chart and thermometer without any instructions or guidance on their use will be worse than useless. If, on top of that, the clinic shows no interest in the chart whatsoever, it is hardly surprising that this can be rather demoralizing and stressful. Looked at positively, the charts give much in the way of information. They show the dates of periods, the frequency of intercourse, the timing of ovulation and the length of the second phase of the cycle between ovulation and the start of the next period (the so-called 'luteal phase'). You can also add onto the chart information about the quality of your cervical mucus during the 'fertile phase' of the cycle and the results of ovulation prediction tests.

Instructions from the hospital about when to take fertility drugs and the results of relevant hormone assays can be added to the chart as well. The chart can, therefore, become a detailed interesting diary of your cycle without it becoming an obsession. It also helps you to see what is going on month by month.

It is of course essential that you are able to read a thermometer. Ideally, a 'fertility' thermometer should be used: this has extra wide degree markings, usually in degrees Celsius. It takes no more than five minutes to teach the average person how to read a thermometer with accuracy and then to record the temperature onto the chart. Usually the surgery nurse or even the chemist will be only too pleased to help teach you how to read your thermometer. If you should turn out to be one of the few who for some reason or other are unable to read a thermometer at all, then you might consider purchasing one of the newer digital thermometers which actually prints out the temperature onto a screen.

The quality of the temperature chart is also important. The best charts take the form of a display sheet making up six cycles. Day one of each chart is the first day of the period. The number of days of bleeding are then recorded and the dates are entered onto the chart. Every morning when you wake up, before you get out of bed, or have a cup of tea or a cuddle, your first waking action (while holding your husband off with one hand) is to reach for the thermometer, place the silver end under your tongue for approximately three minutes and then put the thermometer down. There is no need to read it straight away as the thermometer will stay at its reading for ever. It will only go up if your room catches fire or you unwisely stir your cup of tea with it — when it will explode! It will only go down when you shake it down. So you can record the temperature when you are wide awake or, if you forget, even when you return from work in the evening. Once you have recorded the reading, shake the thermometer down to below 36 degrees, clean it using an antiseptic or cold water (*not* hot water) and then replace it by the bedside ready for the next day. Don't leave it in the bathroom, because if you have to get up to get it, that physical activity can put your resting temperature up. Obviously, if you have to make a frantic dash to the loo, go ahead and then take your temperature later, indicating on the chart that it may not be accurate as a 'resting' temperature.

Each day your temperatures are recorded on the chart and then joined together to form a graph. As an example, it can be seen from Chart 1, that on day 29 (5th May), this patient's temperature was just

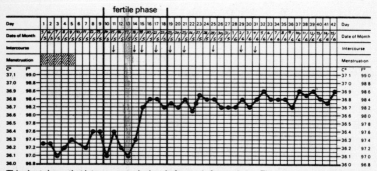

This chart shows that ovulation occurred on day 12. Unfortunately, intercourse did not take place during the fertile phase. The temperature fell and a period occurred.

This chart shows that intercourse took place before and after ovulation. The temperature remained raised and a period did not occur, showing the features of pregnancy. A pregnancy test would be positive when the temperature had remained raised for four weeks.

over 36.2°C. She then started a period changing what had begun as day 29 into her new day 1. The date and temperature have, therefore, been transferred to the beginning of Chart 2. Each chart represents a cycle from day 1 until the next period commences when a new chart is begun.

Chart 1 shows that ovulation occurred on day 12. Unfortunately, intercourse did not take place during the fertile phase. The temperature fell and a period occurred.

This next chart shows that intercourse took place before and after ovulation. The temperature remained raised and a period did not occur, showing the features of pregnancy. A pregnancy test would be positive when the temperature had remained raised for three weeks.

It can be seen from Chart 1 that there has been a fall in temperature on day 12 followed by a rise, after which the temperature remains raised until just before the next period commences. The fall and subsequent rise in temperature represents ovulation. As shown in Figure 8, when ovulation has occurred, the corpus luteum in the ovary produces the hormone progesterone. Progesterone levels go up after ovulation and then fall just before a period. The temperature chart is really a simple way of plotting the changes in progesterone output because the resting body temperature will rise a few 10ths of a degree when ovulation has taken place following the rise in progesterone. So if a chart does not show a significant and sustained temperature rise during the two weeks before the next period commences, ovulation has probably not occurred. Had it done so, the production of progesterone would have led to a corresponding rise in temperature.

Now it is all very well to look in retrospect at Chart 1 and say that day 12-13 was the time of ovulation. But it is certainly not that easy when you are recording the chart from day to day and you gradually see the pattern of the chart unfold. I have, therefore, taken the first part of Chart 2 and broken it down (below) to show what that person would have seen each day as the chart developed. For a 28-day cycle I generally advise that any fall of temperature after day 10 should be acted on and certainly you should act on any subsequent temperature rise. You can, therefore, make use of the chart to go egg-hunting, by timing intercourse with the probable time of ovulation.

A single, lonely episode of intercourse once in mid-cycle is a bit hit-and-miss. You must regard the egg as being rather like a moving target. If only one missile is aimed at it, that missile will probably miss. A salvo of six has a much better chance of making contact! So machine gun tactics are necessary! The time of ovulation really needs to be 'peppered' with intercourse! Now this is where problems can arise for you both — if you let them, e.g. You may feel that 'tonight's the night!' because it's day 12 and this morning there was a fall in temperature. On telling your partner, he may not appreciate the cold-blooded nature of your plans and may feel that he would rather watch the snooker. After persuasion, threats, tears (a little 'come-hither'

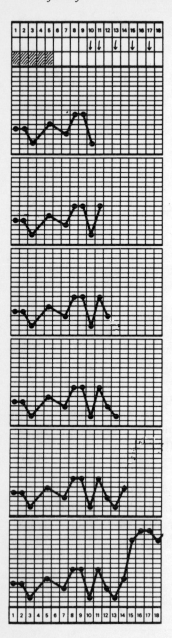

There was a fall in temperature on day 10. This could have been ovulation and intercourse was worthwhile.

The temperature had risen slightly. They were 'in the mood' and tried again.

The temperature fell on day 12. They decided to await events.

By the further fall in temperature they now knew that day 10 was not ovulation, because if it had been, the temperature would have been up by now. So they tried again.

The rise on day 14 was not particularly helpful. It just looked like another zig on a zag.

The subsequent temperature rise on days 15 and 16 showed that the dip on day 13 was ovulation. Further intercourse would be helpful.

Chart 2, stage by stage

seems to work best), your unwilling stud turns off the TV and grumbles up the stairs muttering about the nasty things he would like to do to the chart in particular and to the world in general. But worse is still to come. The temperature goes up and you sit there watching it every day literally praying that it will not come down and so herald the next period's arrival. It does. The whole depressing cycle of events begins again.

Chart watching is dangerous if you let it become too important. The chart does *not* represent a set of rules and orders that must be obeyed. It is, after all, only a piece of paper and intercourse is meant to be fun! You are not having intercourse for the sake of your doctor or because a clinic said so! You really are meant to enjoy it! Whenever I see a patient who is living around her chart too much, I generally stop treatment for a few cycles to give her a break. On returning to charts afterwards, her perspective is restored and she makes sure that she does not fall into the same trap again.

Ideally, the temperature rise after ovulation should be maintained for at least 11 days to give a fertilized egg a chance to implant. A shorter luteal phase may provide a clue to the cause of your infertility.

You should not worry if your own charts are nothing like the examples given. This could indicate that an ovulation disorder is responsible for your infertility and this can usually be corrected.

Hormone assays

Chapter one went into some detail on how the different hormones interacted between the brain, pituitary gland and the ovaries in order to bring about the complex event of ovulation. The chief hormones involved are follicle stimulating hormone (FSH), luteinizing hormone (LH), oestrogen, and progesterone. Another pituitary hormone called prolactin can interfere with the normal production of FSH by the pituitary gland. The male hormone testosterone is also normally produced in small quantities by the female. Just a slight increase in testosterone production can interfere with normal fertility. Disorders of the adrenal glands and thyroid gland can also affect fertility.

If you have an irregular menstrual cycle, or if your periods have stopped altogether, your Infertility Clinic will certainly wish to measure these particular hormones. The hormone levels may indicate the cause of your infertility problem and lead to further investigation and treatment. It can save a considerable amount of time if the Clinic can be presented with the results of these hormone assays on referral by your doctor and the majority of doctors have access to a hospital laboratory which is able to carry out these tests.

If your cycle is a regular one, it should mean that ovulation is a relatively regular and predictable event. While the BBT chart can indicate whether or not you are ovulating, it is now normal practice to measure the actual progesterone level mid-way between ovulation and the start of the next period. This will usually fall on day 21 for a normal 28-day cycle (Fig. 11). This simply involves your doctor taking a blood sample on the appropriate day and sending the sample to the laboratory. When a period begins, the date for the blood test can be easily worked out. If day 21 happens to fall at a week-end, it is perfectly reasonable to delay the test to day 22 or 23. A normal day 21 progesterone level (a measurement of more than 30 nmol per litre) will confirm that ovulation has occurred in that particular cycle. A low progesterone level will mean that ovulation has probably not occurred as there has been an insufficient production of hormone by the ovary. The reason for this may be that the ovary has not been adequately stimulated by FSH and LH from the pituitary.

The similarity in shape between the BBT chart and the above diagram showing the normal progesterone output by the ovary is quite obvious. The BBT chart and progesterone assays complement one another in a practical way too; e.g. it can sometimes be seen from

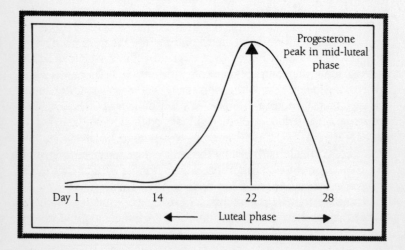

Fig. 11: *Progesterone output during the normal menstrual cycle.*

the chart that a low progesterone level is due to the test having been taken too early in that particular cycle as ovulation (as shown by the temperature rise) was later than expected.

Semen analysis

The semen analysis or 'sperm count' is the basic test of male fertility. Usually this test can easily be arranged by your family doctor. You should be provided with two sets of pathology forms and pots, sufficient for two samples to be tested. It is important to check when the laboratory can do the tests because some hospitals will only carry out sperm counts on a particular day. Laboratories will vary in their instructions but it is now generally accepted that it is sufficient to abstain from ejaculation for just 24 hours before producing the sample. The date and time that the sample is produced must be entered onto both the pathology form and the pot containing the sample. Now most laboratories open at 9.00 am so it is best not to produce your sample much before 8.00 am. If you normally leave for work at 6.00 am, you will simply have to find some excuse (the dentist?) to arrive for work later than usual that day. The sperm sample is produced by masturbation directly into the container, a difficult and sometimes hilarious exercise — you can, however, have fun together doing it! The sample should not be produced by the withdrawal method at intercourse as it is liable to be incomplete. Nor can the sample simply be transferred from the normal condom, because these are usually lubricated with a powerful spermicide. For those of you who have difficulty, however, it is now possible to obtain special condoms which are spermicide-free so that the semen sample can be transferred directly from the condom into the sterile container. (Do *not* send the condom in the pot! The laboratories will make their objections known!) It is essential that the pot is sterile. The pots that have been provided by your doctor have been supplied to the surgery by the hospital and will already be sterile. Do *not* attempt to clean it out first because most detergents and antiseptics are excellent spermicides and will be lethal to the sperm sample. Whoever takes the sample to the laboratory must keep the container warm en route. Sperm are susceptible to cold shock and die rapidly when the temperature falls. So, while in transit, keep the container somewhere warm, in a pocket, under an arm or even down a bra! Essentially, extremes of temperature are to be avoided. (I have had samples produced that have been kept warm in a hot oven or cool in a refrigerator with predictable results.) Don't rely on either surgery transport or Cottage Hospital deliveries to get samples to the laboratory in time. This can often lead to several hours delay in getting samples delivered. Make sure that you know exactly where to take the sample. It is worth the time and effort to take it there yourself.

When the semen sample arrives in the laboratory it will be examined by a trained technician. The following information should be available after the examination:

1. Time interval between production of sample and testing.
2. Appearance of sample.
3. Volume in millilitres (ml).
4. Sperm count in millions per ml.
5. Percentage of sperm moving and quality of movement, e.g. good progressive motility or only sluggish motility. Any clumping together of sperm is noted.
6. Percentage of abnormal sperm and types of abnormality seen.
7. Presence of white blood cells.

A 'normal' sperm count will have the following essential features:

- Volume of 2 ml or more.
- Count greater than 30 million sperm per ml.
- 60 per cent progressive motility within 1 hour of production.
- Less than 30 per cent abnormality rate.
- No white cells present.

(There are further features of the semen analysis and these will be dealt with in the section on male infertility.)

If your semen analysis is less satisfactory than the figures given above, this *may* be a factor in your joint fertility problem, but this does not mean that a pregnancy cannot occur. Indeed, there are many perfectly normal fertile men whose sperm counts, when checked, are surprisingly low. A single poor result in itself is not particularly meaningful as there can be a considerable range from week to week in the same individual. The quality of the semen is almost more important than the count itself, e.g. it would be far preferable to have a sperm count of 15 million per ml with 75 per cent good progressive motility and 25 per cent abnormality rate than a count of 200 million per ml with only 5 per cent sluggish motility and 95 per cent abnormality rate.

It is possible to make rough predictions as to how long it might take for a particular man to get his normally fertile partner pregnant. If the sperm count is 10 million per ml and of good quality, then statistically it can take up to six years to cause a pregnancy. A good quality sperm count of 20 million will take up to three years and 30 million is, of course, within the normal range. If the count is persistently down into single figures, a pregnancy can still occur but it can take a considerable length of time to achieve and it *might* never happen. The above predictions do, however, assume that there is no other infertility factor. Additional infertility problems in your partner do unfortunately make a pregnancy that much more difficult to achieve.

Many couples are referred by their doctors without any baseline investigations having been carried out at all. There is, however, an increasing awareness and interest in infertility problems among doctors. There can be no doubt that to be referred with the following details can often mean that months of frustrating waiting can be avoided, and treatment can be started quickly:

Checklist of routine investigations:

- Rubella screening
- BBT chart for three months
- Hormone profile if cycle is irregular
- Day 21 progesterone assays from two cycles
- Two semen analyses

The Infertility Clinic is the next stop.

4

The Infertility Clinic

If your doctor finds problems indicating that there is a need for further investigation, you will then be referred to see a specialist. Gynaecologists, like all other hospital specialists, receive many types of referrals. These can range from urgent requests to see patients with possible cancer or menstrual haemorrhage, to less urgent routine referrals such as requests for sterilization or investigations into infertility. For *you* the matter is not at all routine and is certainly urgent. The bit that seems to hurt the most is that requests for termination of an unwanted pregnancy are considered to be more urgent than your own referral because of course there is a time-limit in which to perform these operations. In addition, there is such a demand for infertility services, that there is often a delay of several months between your doctor's referral letter and your appointment. The lack of facilities for the adequate treatment of infertility can be so grim, that many couples choose the private sector simply to save waiting time.

Virtually all gynaecologists will see patients who complain of infertility, but not all will be particularly interested in what is to some a fascinating sub-speciality. You do, therefore, have to rely upon your doctor's knowledge about who you should be referred to.

The ideal environment in which to be seen is the Infertility Clinic, where you will see an enthusiastic, informed specialist and the chances are high that it will probably be the same one at each visit. (The main complaint against the routine gynaecology clinic is 'I never see the same doctor twice'.) Investigation and treatment should then follow a logical progression. Infertility Clinics may be 'closed' clinics in that they will only receive referrals from other gynaecologists, or they may have an 'open' referral system with direct access to them by both doctors and hospital specialists. This means that your first appointment may be to see the gynaecologist in the routine clinic first before being referred onwards if your problem is a difficult one.

When you are eventually seen, it is ideal to go as a couple. Gynaecologists always prefer to see both of you even if we know that there is, say, no 'male problem'. There is otherwise always the risk that the partner who attends the clinic is the one who feels 'at fault'. It must be remembered that infertility is never a question of being any individual's 'fault'. You might as well blame yourself for deafness or baldness. Some men are reluctant to attend what they consider is a 'women's clinic', and might take some persuading to come with you. Sometimes this reluctance is due to a fear that they may be found to be lacking in something that may threaten their 'masculinity'. Men have always been good at confusing virility with sterility!

Medical history

It usually takes up to half an hour to take a full infertility history, carry out an examination, explain the findings to you both, and plan on an initial line of investigation and management. Although the history is a very personal one, you should certainly feel no embarrassment over any of the questions you will be asked.

It will help you to have some idea of the typical questions that you will both be asked in the Infertility Clinic and also to explain a gynaecologist's reasons for asking them. For example:

'How old are you both?'

Your ages are obviously very relevant, although much less so for the man than the woman. In Chapter two the relationship between increasing age in the woman and infertility was discussed. If you are in your twenties, time is still on your side even though you might feel that you are becoming ancient! If you are in your late thirties or early forties there is not much time left for you to achieve your goal. When you are in this older age group, it is not simply a matter of getting pregnant. In older age groups, there is a much higher miscarriage rate; there is a greater incidence of Down's Syndrome (although this can be screened for); although you may only *feel* twenty, it is a sad fact of life that you are not, and the body is not as resilient as it was even five years ago. In the older woman, there is a greater chance of complications arising during the pregnancy, especially problems relating to your blood pressure, so there is a high probability that at some stage you would require to be admitted to hospital for rest.

Finally, there is a greater possibility that you will require to have your delivery by Caesarean Section. Some babies in the older woman certainly take some getting!

'For how long have you been married?'

In general, it is not the role of the Infertility Clinic to moralize over whether or not you are legally 'married'. You may even feel that it is none of our business. You want to have a baby and you feel that we should help. In a sense, you are quite right, and we are certainly more concerned to know that the relationship is a happy and stable one. However, for particular treatments, you will find that many clinics will only treat you if you are married, e.g. if you are requesting donor insemination, in-vitro fertilization or GIFT (gamete intrafallopian transfer), or if there is a need to use powerful drugs that may lead to a multiple pregnancy. The reason for this insistence upon marriage is that these treatments can be emotionally very stressful and experience has shown us that a 'married' partnership is better able to withstand the rigours of treatment than if you are technically single. I fully accept that a bit of paper stating that you are married will not keep you together if you don't want to stay with each other, but these guidelines which clinics make for themselves are based upon sound commonsense. At the end of the day there is a baby involved and it has a right to expect two parents and a safe environment.

If you have been living together for only a few months you probably won't have got as far as the Infertility Clinic yet, unless there are pressing reasons why there should be a minimum of delay before you are referred.

'For how long have the two of you been trying to have a baby?'

The length of your relationship is important, but from an infertility point of view, obviously the length of time that you have been trying to start a family within that relationship is more relevant. Normal fertility should result in a pregnancy within two years of trying. However, this does not mean that you need to wait for that long before being seen, especially if you are in an older-than-average age group or if there is a known problem — if, for example, periods are very few and far between.

'Have either of you been trying to have a baby in a previous relationship?'

It is very relevant to know if your infertility precedes this current relationship. If either of you were trying to have a baby with an earlier partner, it is important to know how long you were trying for and whether or not this attempt was successful. If you succeeded in producing a pregnancy with another partner but now cannot do so, there are possible implications. For the woman who has been pregnant before, her secondary infertility may be due to some pelvic inflammation associated with that pregnancy, or possibly her new partner may be infertile; for the man who has fathered children before but now cannot do so, the infertility may be due to some problem with his new partner. However, the fact that he may have already been a father does not necessarily mean that all is well now and that it will be easy for him to repeat this success. If no pregnancy occurred in the earlier relationship, in spite of trying, it would be of some interest to know if your previous partner has since succeeded in being associated with a pregnancy. Such a pregnancy may imply that you have a factor which contributed to the infertility when the two of you were together. Understandably, you might have lost track of your past partners and information relating to their subsequent fertility may not be available.

'Have you ever been pregnant or (in his case) caused a pregnancy before?'

All information relating to previous pregnancies is of importance. What was the outcome of each pregnancy? Was the pregnancy uneventful? Did you go to full term? Was labour induced? Did you have a normal delivery? Were there any post-natal complications? Is the baby alive and well? Is the child still living with both of you?

If you miscarried, or had a termination of pregnancy, how far did the pregnancy progress? Was an evacuation of any retained remnants of the pregnancy (D & C) required? Were you well afterwards? Did you require any antibiotics? The answers to these questions may indicate that infection complicated the previous miscarriage or termination.

'What methods of contraception have you used in the past?'

The relevance of this question is that certain methods of contraception can have infertility consequences. The intra-uterine contraceptive device (the **IUCD** or 'coil') can be associated with pelvic infection. If there is pre-existing pelvic inflammatory disease, the insertion of a foreign body such as an IUCD into the uterus can lead to an acute flare-up of the condition. There is also the possibility that the presence of the device in the uterus could actually lead to an acute pelvic infection. It is chiefly for this reason that gynaecologists are reluctant to insert an IUCD into the uterus of a woman who has not yet had a child.

The standard combined contraceptive Pill works as an efficient contraceptive by suppressing the normal hormonal interaction between the pituitary gland and the ovaries. As a result, the pituitary and ovaries go into a limbo state and egg development and ovulation each cycle does not occur. The menstrual bleed that occurs when you come to the end of each packet is not a natural period but simply what is called a 'withdrawal' bleed when the Pill is stopped for a week between packs. If your menstrual cycle before going onto the Pill was a rather lazy one, with infrequent periods, you may find that when the Pill is stopped, the pituitary and ovaries continue in their state of inactivity. It is not always the case that 'normal service will be resumed as soon as possible'. If you stopped the Pill in order to start your family and your cycle does not rapidly return to normal, you may have to wait many months before you even have an opportunity of becoming pregnant. If you are *not* having periods you will not be ovulating and a pregnancy cannot occur. Fortunately, this condition, known as post-Pill-related-amenorrhoea, is usually fairly easy to correct.

'Have either of you had any serious illnesses or operations?'

This is an enquiry into each of your past medical histories. *All* illnesses, hospital admissions, and operations should be mentioned. An admission to hospital a few years ago with abdominal pain for which no cause could be found, may seem irrelevant to you, but could in fact be highly significant.

A history of a sexually transmitted disease may indicate the possibility of an obstruction of the fallopian tubes which can be a complication of these infections.

The medical and surgical history of the male is also important. Any operations in the scrotal or groin areas can be important factors in infertility. Were there any problems with undescended testicles as a child? If so, was surgery carried out and at what age? Your age at such surgery is important because if the operation was left until puberty or later, then sperm production in that testicle is likely to be severely affected.

'Have either of you been on any regular medication?'

All regular prescriptions of medicines should be mentioned. These may give a clue as to the cause of your infertility. In the male, certain blood pressure lowering drugs and tranquillizers can affect sperm production.

'Do either of you smoke cigarettes or drink alcohol?'

There is no doubt that it is in your joint interests and the interests of your future family that you are both as fit and healthy as possible when conception takes place. Cigarette smoking has been proven to have widespread harmful effects on the body. It is now being achnowledged that the fertility of women who smoke is half that of non-smoking women. It is also generally accepted that smoking in men reduces both the quantity and quality of sperm production (spermatogenesis). Heavy smoking is regarded as 20 cigarettes or more a day, but even 10 a day can lead to problems. If you are trying to have a baby, then you should both stop smoking. If you do succeed in becoming pregnant and continue to smoke heavily, the very high carbon monoxide levels in your unborn baby's blood can impair its growth and development. The message should be loud and clear!

Animal experiments have shown that a moderate alcohol intake by the female at the time of conception can interfere with the normal development of the early embryo and so lead to miscarriage. There is as yet no conclusive evidence that the same effect will occur in the human pregnancy. Certainly, a prolonged alcohol intake during pregnancy can have disastrous effects upon the baby leading to a condition known as fetal alcohol intoxication syndrome. In the male, it is well known that a moderate alcohol intake will reduce both spermatogenesis and the production of the male hormone testosterone. This does not mean that the occasional lager or pint or two of beer will cause problems, but it may do if you are a 4+ pints per day man or if you have a high regular intake of spirits. Very high alcohol abuse, to the point of being drunk, will mean that conception itself may be impossible because the man will be temporarily impotent and be unable to 'rise to the occasion'.

'Have any infertility investigations been carried out yet?'

Hopefully some basic investigations will have already been carried out by the family doctor as outlined in the previous chapter, and the results of these tests will be available to the Infertility Clinic at the time of your consultation. Some couples will have already been extensively investigated elsewhere and are now being referred for more intensive treatment if the problem is proving to be a difficult one. In others, the referral is simply due to the couple having moved away from the area of their own clinic and continuity of infertility treatment has been requested. If this is the case, the Infertility Clinic will need to write to the previous consultant and ask for a relevant summary of past investigations and treatments.

Some couples 'do the rounds' (especially in major cities where there are many consultants) going from specialist to specialist in the hope of finding someone who will help them. Sometimes they can even be under the care of more than one specialist at the same time, so that they receive differing plans of management and become totally confused. This is also a sure way of annoying both consultants when they find out, and they are bound to! You will all be able to understand the anguish and desperation that is experienced when every available treatment has been tried and has failed. Some of you will have been there. In many instances, 'specialist-hopping' is due to impatience with the treatment and advice being given at one clinic, or is due to a friend saying 'You simply *must* go and see Dr . . ., everyone says he is *marvellous!*'

In order to avoid unnecessary repetition of tests, it is important to make sure that the clinic you are currently attending is aware of all past investigations and treatments.

'What are your periods like?'

This question will usually lead on to a whole series of questions relating to your menstrual cycle. You will recall from the last chapter how BBT charts show ovulation occurring about two weeks before the onset of the next period. It is, therefore, very important to establish the pattern that your own cycle takes in order to determine whether or not ovulation is a predictable event. If your cycle is very erratic with periods ranging anywhere between 4-12 weeks apart, this could be an important factor in your infertility. Going to the other extreme, if your cycle is a very short one of less than 21 days, then ovulation is unlikely to be occurring normally.

If periods have stopped altogether (secondary amenorrhoea), you will be asked about any major change in your lifestyle. A crash diet leading to a dramatic weight loss is well recognized as being able to cause periods to stop, a condition known as weight-loss-related-amenorrhoea. Regaining a few pounds is often all that it takes to restore your cycle to normal. (It is interesting to note that women athletes of international standard who have trained themselves to be at the peak of physical fitness, nearly all have absent periods. If they want to have a period they simply train a little less vigorously!)

You will be asked about the number of days of bleeding you have with each period and about the heaviness of the blood loss. This is relevant because very prolonged and heavy periods can be caused by conditions such as fibroids in the uterus (non-malignant tumours of muscle and fibrous tissue) or another troublesome condition called endometriosis. Both fibroids and endometriosis, apart from causing distressingly unpleasant periods, can also lead to infertility.

The amount of pain (dysmenorrhoea) that you experience with periods will also be of interest to the clinic. If periods are completely painless, this may indicate that ovulation is not occurring. (A similar situation occurs in women who are prescribed the contraceptive Pill. The Pill prevents ovulation from occurring and the withdrawal bleed that follows the end of each packet is usually painless.) In cycles where ovulation is occurring, it is normal to have at least some discomfort during the first day or two of bleeding. If the dysmenorrhoea is severe, it may indicate that there is some pelvic disease such as endometriosis causing both the pain and the infertility.

You will be asked if you have any bleeding between your periods. It is quite common for a little spotting to occur at mid-cycle at the time of ovulation. Haphazard bleeding occurring at any time in the cycle, or, for example after intercourse, may mean that there is a minor problem with the cervix of the uterus, such as a cervical polyp or 'erosion', or perhaps even polyps within the uterus itself. These conditions are straightforward to treat.

'Are you aware of the fertile phase of the cycle when you are most likely to become pregnant?'

Many couples have got no idea at all of the best time in each cycle to try for a baby. Never feel too embarrassed to say you don't know. Some people think that they do know, but on further enquiry we can get some very surprising answers! I have frequently been told by women that they think that the best time to conceive is immediately after a period is finished or just before the next period is due. It's not that they are stupid, they simply do not know. Sometimes they have received misguided though well-meaning advice from a friend.

'Taking an average week, how many times a week do you think that you are having intercourse?'

It seems obvious to say that intercourse must be taking place for a pregnancy to occur. Many infertile couples have such infrequent intercourse that it is hardly surprising that a pregnancy does not happen. Sometimes the lack of intercourse is due to overwork and tiredness, or simply that it is no longer fun and has become a mechanical, unhappy, and boring event, associated always with their infertility. Some couples hope that if intercourse only takes place during ovulation, the sperm count will have built up during their abstinence and so increase their chances of success. Well, this is partly true, in that the actual sperm count will be higher, but the motility of the sperm may be reduced. I can vividly recall a couple who had experienced ten years of primary infertility, and who had religiously followed the advice of a neighbour and only had intercourse once a month. This was always on the wrong day of the cycle, and only took place once each month because they were worried when they were told that more frequent intercourse might result in twins. Sad but true.

Other couples have intercourse every day. While enjoyable and worthy of admiration, they may also be going 'into the red' and be depleting their own personal sperm-bank of its stock.

'Do you have any pain or discomfort with intercourse?'

This is an important question for two reasons. First of all, as already mentioned, intercourse is meant to be fun and not a painful experience. Pain at penetration may be due to the vaginal entrance being insufficiently stretched. Sometimes pain is due to inadequate lubrication perhaps because foreplay has been too hasty or inadequate. Once you know that intercourse is going to hurt you, it is only natural that you will tense up your pelvic muscles guaranteeing that it will hurt again. Deep pelvic pain at intercourse can sometimes be so acute that it can make you stop (and never want to try again!) Deep pain may be due to endometriosis affecting the ovaries or pelvic ligaments. Characteristically, endometriosis results in painful, heavy periods, pain on intercourse and infertility. Another important cause of deep pelvic pain is pelvic inflammatory disease (PID). The tubes and ovaries may be stuck down in the pelvis. If the ovaries are stuck down by adhesions from previous infection and are now close to the upper vagina, they can literally be thumped 20 times a minute during intercourse. Now the ovaries have the same nerve supply as the testicles. See how a man reacts at the mere *thought* of having this happen to his testicles during intercourse!

'Have you noticed any vaginal discharge?'

It is completely normal for there to be some discharge from the vagina. It should be clear white, have a non-offensive odour and there should be no itching or irritation. If the discharge is very profuse, it may just be a variation of the normal, but if it is associated with itching there is usually some infection present. The commonest infections are a yeast infection called **candida** ('thrush') and infection with a little organism called **trichomonas**. It is important to treat both these infections as they can interfere with sperm survival. Fortunately, treatment is usually straightforward, although both infections can be difficult to eradicate. It must be remembered that these infections can be passed between both partners, so both of you (this is especially true with trichomonas infections) may require treatment.

Medical examination

After your medical history has been taken, the doctor will wish to examine you. This is not something to dread or to be embarrassed about. Doctors are very aware of the apprehension you may be feeling and the examination is carried out as gently as possible. After all, we do want you to come back again!

You may find that the clinic will wish to weigh you if you are apparently either very underweight or overweight. Examination of the front of the neck is carried out if it appears that the thyroid gland is enlarged. Breast examination is a part of a routine gynaecological examination. Sometimes there is evidence of milk production (galactorrhoea) which may be due to an excess of one of the pituitary hormones, prolactin. A significantly raised prolactin secretion (a condition called hyperprolactinaemia) can cause infertility. This is often associated with irregular, infrequent periods. After further investigation, it is usually easy to bring the prolactin level down and restore fertility to normal.

A careful examination of the abdomen is now carried out. Areas of tenderness are noted, and especially any swellings in the lower abdomen which might be rising up out of the pelvis. Such a swelling might be a fibroid of the uterus or an ovarian cyst. At times it is even a pregnant uterus!

The vaginal or pelvic examination is very important and sometimes most informative. It is also the part of the examination that you might be most frightened about. Remember one thing. Doctors know that if they hurt you, not only will you vigorously protest, but you will react by becoming tense and rigid. It is, therefore, in their interests as well as yours to examine you as gently as possible. The clinic staff will do everything they can to reassure you and help you to relax.

The doctor wears a lubricated glove to carry out the pelvic examination. A check is first made of the entrance to the vagina. Very occasionally at this examination, it can be seen that intercourse with full penetration has never taken place because of a very tight, narrow opening into the vagina. The couple may have been too embarrassed to have offered this information when the history was being taken, or they may have genuinely thought that normal intercourse with penetration was actually occurring. Intercourse is, of course, a normal requirement for a natural conception to occur. Once this problem has been found, it is usually easy to correct and that may be all the treatment that will be required to bring about a subsequent pregnancy.

The vagina itself is now examined and any abnormality noted. There can be rare problems such as a double vagina or cysts in the vaginal wall.

The uterus is assessed at this stage of the internal examination. The normal uterus, tubes and ovaries cannot be felt by just examining the lower abdomen. The uterus can only just be felt abdominally when it reaches the size of a 12-week pregnancy. The examination of the uterus is carried out by two fingers placed in the vagina behind the cervix which lift the uterus up so that it is also felt by the other hand which is placed on the lower abdomen. Between the two hands, the size, shape and mobility of the uterus can be determined. An enlarged, irregularly shaped uterus probably means that there are fibroids present. It is impossible to tell by this examination whether or not the fibroids may be distorting the cavity of the uterus or by virtue of their size be compressing and obstructing the tubes. If there is any undue tenderness, this may indicate the presence of pelvic inflammation. A uterus that is fixed solidly in its position and immobile could imply that there is scarring from endometriosis. (Fibroids and endometriosis are dealt with in Chapter seven.)

The cervix is the only part of the uterus that can be seen as well as felt, because it protrudes into the upper part of the vagina. The normal cervix should feel smooth and regular and be of adequate length. The opening into the canal of the cervix should not be too distorted by lacerations from a previous delivery. In order to inspect the cervix, a lubricated instrument called a speculum is gently inserted into the vagina. (On a cold day you can only hope that the metal speculum has been warmed first!) An excellent view of the cervix is obtained. If the preliminary history reveals that you have a vaginal discharge indicating that specimen swabs should be taken for culture, or that a cervical smear is required, then the speculum examination will be carried out before the full pelvic examination in order to perform these tests.

It is not usually necessary to examine your partner at this stage, unless it is apparent that there is a significant male infertility factor. (See Chapter eight.)

When the full history and examination have been completed, you will find that your infertility places you both into one of three broad categories, although there may be some overlap:

1. There is nothing specific in either of your medical histories or on examination. At this stage your infertility is unexplained.
2. Your menstrual cycle is so erratic that ovulation, even if it is occurring at all, will be completely unpredictable.
3. Your history and examination suggest that there may be damage to the fallopian tubes and this may account for your infertility.

The specialist will now explain his findings to you and outline the steps to be taken to further investigate and treat you. Depending upon the investigations that your doctor may have already had carried out, it is sometimes possible to start specific treatment at your first attendance at the Infertility Clinic. If there are any essential investigations such as Rubella screening that must be obtained before treatment can begin, then the clinic will of course carry out this test as quickly as possible. You will find that investigation and treatment will go hand in hand. Apart from Rubella screening which comes first, none of the investigations are carried out in any particularly rigid order. It will depend very much upon the category you fall into. If your infertility seems to be unexplained at your initial visit, then all the basic tests will be carried out. If menstrual irregularity is the chief apparent problem, then after hormone assays, treatment will be given to regulate and stimulate ovulation. Should your history and examination point to a possible tubal problem, then a specific test of tubal patency (to check whether or not the tubes are blocked) will be carried out as an early investigation, rather than initially giving the tubes the benefit of the doubt.

Your specialist will outline the plan of investigation and treatment to you. It is very important that you fully understand what you are being told. You must ask for further explanation if there is anything that you do not fully understand.

Hopefully, you will both be able to leave the clinic with some new optimism.

5

Special investigations

Hopefully, the basic tests of Rubella screening, BBT charts, progesterone assays, and semen analyses will have been set up by your doctor. If not, they will be rapidly carried out by the Infertility Clinic. There are, however, a number of additional investigations that may be required.

The post-coital test

While it is obviously essential to know the detailed analysis of your partner's semen, it is equally vital to know how his sperm will behave after they have been ejaculated into the vagina at intercourse. In Chapter one, it was explained how the vaginal acidity is very hostile to sperm and how their survival depends upon their ability to reach the alkaline mucus of the cervical canal. The post-coital test (PCT) assesses exactly that. It is in fact a simple form of compatability testing.

An appointment is made for you to attend the clinic as close as possible to the estimated time of your ovulation. It is at this time of the cycle that cervical mucus is particularly receptive to sperm. Under the influence of an increasing production of oestrogen by the ovary, the mucus becomes very profuse, clear and easily flowing, very similar in fact to saliva. You may yourself notice an increase in this mucus secretion from the vagina at this time of the cycle.

When you are actually in the cycle during which the test is to be carried out, it is worthwhile to check the timing of your appointment once your period has begun. The reason for this is that the appointment will probably have been made several weeks in advance and the date will have been determined from your cycle length and previous

BBT charts. It is, therefore, quite common to find that the appointment date has been made for the wrong time of the cycle because of unpredictable variations in the length of cycles since your previous clinic visit. In that case, simply contact the clinic as early as possible after the beginning of your period. Usually it is a simple matter for them to rearrange your test for the correct day of the cycle.

You will have been asked to have had intercourse several hours earlier, not just an hour or two before your clinic appointment. This usually means intercourse the night before for a morning clinic and early that morning for an afternoon clinic, which means that your partner will then need to stagger off to work. It's not always easy to have intercourse on demand because a doctor has requested it for a particular test. For many couples it does tend to make everything very clinical, a complete 'turn-off' from what should normally be a loving and enjoyable event. For some couples, the clinical background to the test can make intercourse impossible and some men may even fail to have an erection. This in turn simply leads to more tension and worry about what the clinic will say, and fears that they may be thought to be wasting the clinic's time. You need have no fear of this as the clinic staff are only too aware of the possible difficulties. The only way around the problem is for you to inject some fun back into love-making! Suspenders and stocking-tops, or a trail of clothing up the stairs with a little note saying 'I'm all yours . . . if you can find me!', will usually have at least an interesting effect on a partner's flagging interests!

On being seen at the clinic, a general updating of information is made, such as the assessing of BBT charts and progesterone assays. You will be asked how long ago you last had intercourse and usually this will be anywhere from 6 to 12 hours earlier. Having intercourse just an hour before the test is carried out is not particularly helpful to you or to the clinic. First of all it means that you've probably been in a frantic rush or else that you've had intercourse in the hospital car park! Secondly, there has not really been a sufficient lapse of time to adequately assess sperm survival in the cervical mucus.

In order to perform a post-coital test, the cervix is examined with a speculum as described in the last chapter. In just a few seconds, and quite painlessly, mucus is drawn up out of the canal of the cervix and placed upon a clean slide. While this is being done the 'stretchability' of the mucus is assessed (Fig. 12).

The mucus on the slide is then covered with a glass coverslip and examined under the microscope.

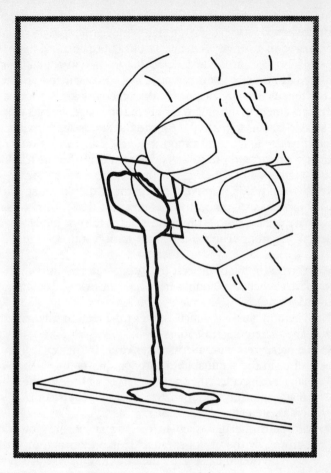

Fig. 12: Glass coverslip 'stretching' mucus on slide.

A post-coital test is positive and completely normal when the mucus is found to be very 'stretchable', and contains many sperm. These sperm must on the whole be normal in appearance and be moving vigorously across the slide, not simply shaking on the spot. There will always be some sperm seen that are abnormal in their shape and either not moving at all, or at best only very sluggishly. Motility is graded from '0' for dead sperm to '4' for vigorously forward-moving sperm. Under high magnification, a perfect post-coital test will have at least 20 grade 4 progressively motile sperm present in every area examined on the slide. Indeed, sometimes the sperm are present in such numbers that the slide can actually look like a neat sperm sample, rather than a mucus sample.

When a good positive post-coital test has been obtained, it implies that the sperm count is satisfactory, that the sperm are sufficiently motile to be able to reach the cervical canal and that there is no major cervical mucus hostility factor that may otherwise kill the sperm off. Sperm movement in the mucus is only the first stage of a long journey. The second stage is to reach the egg and the third stage to get into the egg and fertilize it. If sperm cannot generate sufficient movement to produce good forward progression in good mucus they are less likely to be able to penetrate the egg.

A post-coital test is negative if no sperm or only dead sperm are seen in the mucus. Although a negative test does not necessarily imply that there is a serious problem, it can be the first indication that something is wrong. The main reasons for a negative test are:

- Incorrect timing of the test (e.g. too late in the cycle).
- A cycle where ovulation is not occurring (a so-called **anovulatory cycle**).
- Thick and glue-like mucus rather than clear and flowing.
- A low or zero sperm count.
- The presence of sperm antibodies either in the cervical mucus itself or in the seminal fluid carrying the sperm.
- A failure to ejaculate the sperm into the vagina (e.g. where there is major difficulty with penetration at intercourse or problems such as premature ejaculation).
- The sperm are deposited in the vagina but are unwittingly destroyed by the use of spermicide in a lubricant, or washed away with douching because the patient wants to make herself 'clean' for the clinic.

If the post-coital test is negative, the next step is to repeat it. If the test remains negative when carried out at the correct time of the cycle and where the semen analysis is known to be normal, then additional tests are required.

Sperm invasion test

If your post-coital tests are repeatedly negative in spite of good quality mucus and normal sperm counts, it is going to be important to find out what is actually taking place when sperm and mucus come into contact with each other. An appointment is made exactly as for a post-coital test at the estimated time of ovulation. This time you are asked *not* to have intercourse for the previous 24 hours, but to bring with you, in a specially provided container, a semen sample produced in the previous hour. Remember to keep the sample warm en route to the clinic. It is also important on your arrival that the clinic staff are aware of the fact that you are there with a fresh sperm sample for a sperm invasion test so as to avoid any undue delay. From your point of view, the whole procedure is very similar to the post-coital test, in that a sample of mucus is withdrawn from the canal of the cervix. The mucus is placed onto a glass slide and a drop of semen from the container is placed next to it. When the glass cover slip is placed carefully on the slide, the surfaces of the mucus and semen come into contact with each other. (The remainder of the semen sample is not wasted but artificially introduced into and around the cervical canal.) The slide is now examined under the microscope. On inspecting the semen side of the slide, a general impression of sperm density and motility is obtained. Sometimes areas of sperm 'clumping' are noted which had not been commented upon before by laboratory staff when semen analyses were being carried out. These clumped sperm usually mean that there is an antibody present in your partner's seminal fluid which is sticking his sperm together.

Attention is now focused on the area where the sperm and mucus meet. In a normal sperm invasion test, during the course of the next quarter of an hour, the motile sperm will mass along this line of contact and rather like advancing columns of troops, will penetrate into the territory of the mucus. with whip-like movements of their tail-sections, the sperm continue to move forward through the mucus.

However, sometimes this penetration is only minimal before the sperm are stopped literally dead in their tracks. The initial progressive grade 4 motility slows down to a 'shaking-on-the-spot' grade 1 motility and finally to zero. While such a result will explain why the earlier post-coital tests were negative, it does not in itself indicate whether the fault lies with the sperm or the mucus.

There is, therefore, a refinement of the sperm invasion test called a '**cross-over sperm invasion test**'. This test assesses the ability of your partner's sperm to penetrate known normal mucus, and of known normal sperm to penetrate your mucus. In addition to this, a blood sample from each of you, together with a semen and mucus sample, are sent for sperm antibody tests. In this way, it is possible to find out whether the negative post-coital test is due to an antibody or some other factor in your mucus or your partner's semen.

Further hormone assays

Basic hormone assays may have already been carried out through your doctor (Chapter 3). It is very useful to have a few day 21 progesterone assays carried out if you have a reasonably regular 28-day cycle. If the result is above 30 nmol per litre and corresponds with the luteal phase of the cycle as shown on your temperature charts, then this confirms biochemically that ovulation is occurring in that particular cycle. I have already mentioned how BBT charts and day 21 progesterone assays complement each other. The BBT charts below demonstrate this.

The first chart below shows a normal 28-day cycle with a very satisfactory day 21 progesterone level of 72 nmol per litre. The chart and the progesterone level correlate well with each other.

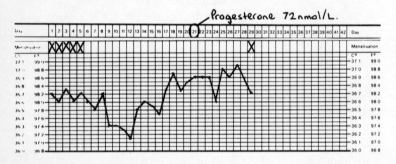

The second chart shows that the day 21 progesterone level is very adequate at 68 nmol per litre, but the length of the luteal phase and the duration of temperature rise are insufficient to allow implantation to occur even if the egg was fertilized.

There is, however, little point in having a day 21 progesterone assay carried out if your cycle is very erratic, because the test will probably have been taken too early in the cycle.

The next chart demonstrates how a routine day 21 progesterone assay of only 1.3 nmol per litre could be misleading unless a BBT chart has been kept as well. This particular cycle was longer than usual with ovulation being delayed and only occurring on day 23. If the BBT

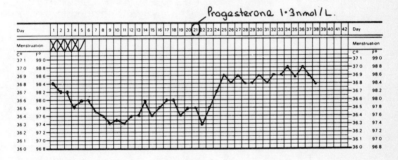

chart was not being kept as well it could easily have been assumed from the blood test alone that this woman had not ovulated that cycle.

Many infertility clinics will now routinely carry out a hormone profile, but this becomes especially important if your cycle is irregular and your periods are becoming further apart.

As explained earlier, the major hormones involved in egg production are FSH, LH, oestrogen and progesterone. In addition to these, the other hormones that may play a part are the male hormone **testosterone** (usually only present at low levels in women), another pituitary hormone called **prolactin** and **thyroxine** from the thyroid gland.

The commonest disorder which affects ovulation is a condition known as **Polycystic Ovary Disease (PCOD)**. It is due essentially to a slight over-production of male hormone by the adrenal glands that sit on top of the kidneys. The upshot of this is that this excess of male hormone is converted in body fat to oestrogen. This in turn leads to a disturbance in the normal production of FSH and LH. Much more LH than FSH is produced which stimulates the ovaries to become packed full of many tiny cysts (hence the word polycystic which means many cysts) which represent immature egg follicles.

Characteristically, patients with PCOD usually have longer intervals between their periods (**oligomenorrhoea**), and may be overweight. Their hormone profiles show a high level of LH compared to FSH, at levels greater than three to one. The level of male hormone, testosterone, is often also moderately raised.

The pituitary hormone prolactin is the hormone responsible for milk production after having a baby. Sometimes there is an over-production of this hormone, a condition called **hyperprolactin-aemia**. Oligomenorrhoea often results accompanied by milk secretion by the breasts.

The infertility that is associated with irregular ovulation patterns, PCOD, hyperprolactinaemia, and thyroid disorders, can often be successfully treated and will be dealt with in the following chapter. Very occasionally the ovaries 'run out of eggs' much earlier than expected. This leads to a state of **ovarian failure** or **premature menopause** ('change of life'). A pregnancy in such couples is still possible but only by means of an egg donation from another patient, an option that will be discussed in Chapter nine.

Ultrasonography

Ultrasound scanning was first developed for use in obstetrics to investigate and monitor the well-being and growth of the fetus. Ultrasound technology has developed rapidly and it is now possible to follow the growth of an egg follicle throughout the cycle. Ovarian scanning plays an important part in infertility management, chiefly in checking that normal development of the follicle (or follicles) is taking place and that ovulation is occurring. This 'tracking' of the follicle can be of great value when a particular treatment such as artificial insemination is being carried out, in order to pinpoint ovulation with greater accuracy.

Accurate assessment of follicular growth is essential for complex assisted conception techniques such as in-vitro fertilization. Here, ultrasound is used not only to monitor the growth of the follicles, but the actual egg removal from the follicle is carried out using ultrasound-directed and -guided techniques rather than surgery (Chapter nine).

Endometrial biopsy

The lining endometrium of the uterus undergoes changes during each cycle. When ovulation has taken place, there is an increase in progesterone production and the endometrium becomes thickened in preparation for the possible implantation of a fertilized egg. The cells of this 'secretory' endometrium show characteristic changes when examined under the microscope.

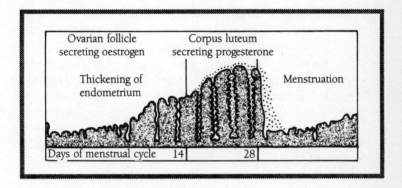

Fig. 13: The endometrium at the various stages of the menstrual cycle.

If progesterone output is inadequate, development of the endometrium may not be sufficiently advanced to allow implantation to take place. A specimen or biopsy of the endometrium will indicate whether or not its stage of development is in phase with the stage of the cycle. If there is more than a two-day lag between these stages of the cycle and endometrium, this may indicate that there is an inadequate production of progesterone.

The biopsy is timed to be taken 2-3 days before the period is due. It can be carried out in the Infertility Clinic itself without any preliminary preparation or anaesthetic. You are placed in a special examination chair and a speculum examination of the cervix is carried out as explained earlier. A fine suction curette is passed gently into the cavity of the uterus via the cervix. In this way fragments of endometrium are obtained for examination. At the most you may experience some slight discomfort.

Some clinics may wish to carry out an endometrial biopsy as a matter of routine. Its value in general infertility management is, however, limited. When secretory endometrium is found, this indicates that ovulation has occurred but the test only gives information for that particular cycle. A combination of BBT charts, progesterone assays, and ultrasound will give a much better assessment regarding the normality of ovulation. (If tuberculosis (an infection that can affect the uterus and tubes) is suspected, a full curettage under a general anaesthetic just before the period is due is required in order to obtain sufficient endometrium for TB culture.)

Ovulation prediction

When your cycle is regular, ovulation is probably going to be a fairly predictable event, the variation of ovulation timing each cycle ranging from 1-3 days. You might notice an increase in cervical mucus at this stage in your cycle which can be a very precise indicator that ovulation is imminent. Cycles which are of variable lengths are more of a problem. BBT charts will indicate when you might be ovulating, but you will not know for sure until after the temperature rise. By using the BBT chart correctly and acting on the dips and the subsequent temperature rise, you are unlikely to miss ovulation, but this does depend upon your being able to have regular intercourse at this time. Both BBT charts and progesterone assays give only retrospective evidence of ovulation. Ovarian ultrasound and follicle tracking will give information about follicle growth and will suggest when ovulation might be imminent. But even ultrasound can only confirm ovulation after the event when the follicle will be seen to be empty. Another problem is that ultrasound scanning is time-consuming and it is not a practical procedure to carry out in every cycle. Furthermore, ultrasound facilities are not going to be universally available when required at every clinic.

Wouldn't it be useful to know for sure that you were going to ovulate in the next 24 hours? The signal that ovulation is going to occur within that time is the surge of LH that occurs just prior to ovulation (Figs. 7 and 8). Until recently, the only way of detecting the LH surge was by sophisticated laboratory assays. It is now possible to purchase ovulation predictor kits as a DIY method of detecting the LH surge yourself at home. These kits can be bought over the counter in chemist shops; you don't need a prescription. Take advice on which one to buy because some are simpler to use than others. They are also rather expensive, although with some kits cheaper refill kits are available. To avoid wasting your money, it is in your interests that you carefully follow the clear instructions that are given with the kit and carry out the 1-7 days of testing at the correct time of your cycle.

The test detects the LH surge in an early morning urine sample with remarkable accuracy. A specially designed dip-stick is used each day and this changes colour when exposed to increasing levels of LH in your urine sample. The colour change is easy to detect and indicates that ovulation is likely to occur in the next 24 hours. Intercourse during this time may be very worthwhile.

If you are keeping a BBT chart it would be both useful and interesting to record the day of the colour change on the chart and then to observe the timing of the subsequent temperature rise.

Predictor kits do not suit everyone. It has been said that they are an expensive way of keeping a temperature chart. I don't think that verdict is entirely fair, because it does at least give prospective information. Certainly many women enjoy having more insight into how their body is working. If your cycle has always been very regular and ovulation has always been predictable and confirmed in the past with good day 21 progesterone assays, then you probably don't need either BBT charts or predictor kits. Simply keep a note of when the fertile phase of your cycle is likely to be and enjoy it!

Tubal patency tests

This test checks whether or not your tubes are in a fully open state. Healthy fallopian tubes are an essential requirement in order for a pregnancy to occur naturally. The tubes are the pathways that permit the ascending sperm to reach the egg, and then allow the embryo to reach the uterus for implantation. As already mentioned in Chapter one they are complex structures which not only assist in the transport of the sperm and egg, but provide the ideal environment for fertilization to occur and are then able to sustain the early embryo. The outer fimbrial end of the tube has a very intimate relationship with the ovary and thereby increases the otherwise random chance of 'picking up' an egg. The fine hairs or cilia in the ampulla of the tube beat towards the uterus and set up a propulsive current in that direction. In contrast, a countercurrent of contraction waves arises from the isthmus (narrowing) of the tube close to the uterus, moving outwards towards the ampulla, thereby assisting sperm transport towards the egg. Once the egg has been fertilized, the early embryo is nourished by the fluid environment within the tube which provides it with an essential energy source.

The tubes are, essentially, extremely delicate structures and easily damaged. If infection has caused damage to the cilia-bearing cells, without obstructing the tube, a fertilized egg may be inadequately propelled towards the uterus and become trapped within the tube as an ectopic pregnancy. If both tubes are completely obstructed then sperm will be unable to have access to the egg and fertilization cannot occur. But the egg too must have access to the tube. If the ovaries are covered with adhesion (tissue that can result from previous inflammation or surgery), then such access will be prevented.

The major cause of tubal damage and adhesion formation is infection. The infection may have arisen following a miscarriage or termination of pregnancy or even following a completely normal pregnancy. Sexually transmitted infections may have led to pelvic inflammatory disease. Pelvic tuberculosis is not uncommon among communities who are exposed to this disease. Tubal damage can be caused by other infections close to the tubes and ovaries: peritonitis, for example, arising from appendicitis. Surgery within the pelvis can itself lead to damaging adhesion formation around the tubes and ovaries. Infection and subsequent adhesions can occur without any apparent episode of ill-health; perhaps even viral infections in childhood can cause silent damage which only becomes apparent years later when infertility occurs. Lastly, there are always women who have voluntarily had their tubes blocked by being sterilized. For a variety of reasons circumstances may have now changed and they bitterly regret having taken such a final step and are desperately seeking to have their fertility restored.

About 15 per cent of all women who attend an Infertility Clinic will have a tubal problem. It is interesting that half of these women will have no past medical history to account for their damaged tubes.

So when should you have your tubes checked? As a generalization, if there is no history suggesting that there might be a tubal problem, it is reasonable, at least initially, to give the tubes the benefit of the doubt. In treating and investigating infertility, it is important to be selective and not blindly carry out every test on every patient. Tubal patency tests can be expensive. For example, if the next 100 patients to attend my Infertility Clinic automatically had a patency test carried out by laparoscopy (a special telescope that allows the doctor to view the interior of the abdominal cavity), regardless of history, the cost to the NHS (excluding the cost of the operation and medical time) would be £30,000 in order to find the 15 patients with a tubal problem. Treatment and investigation often go hand in hand and many women will become pregnant on treatment before any tubal patency test has been carried out. On the other hand, if there is a history suggesting a likely tubal cause for your infertility, then a patency test may very well be one of the first investigations to be suggested to you. Similarly, if you are in an older age group, the state of your tubes will need to be known sooner rather than later. The indications for tubal patency testing are:

- A past history of possible pelvic infection due to peritonitis, appendicitis, pelvic TB, pelvic inflammatory disease or sexually transmitted diseases.
- A history of having had pelvic surgery, e.g. a previous ectopic pregnancy or removal of an ovarian cyst.
- If there is now secondary infertility when there have been no problems in the past in achieving a pregnancy.
- When pregnancy does not occur in spite of all other investigations being completely normal.
- Before carrying out very expensive infertility drug therapy, to ensure that there is at least no tubal cause for the infertility and to thereby justify the expense of such treatment (it would be foolish to spend many hundreds of pounds on a particular treatment and then find that the tubes were blocked).

All tubal patency tests should be carried out during the first half of the cycle so as not to disturb a possible early pregnancy. If the test were to push an early embryo back along the tube towards the ovary, it will have increased in size by the time it has returned to its original position on its journey to the uterus and can get stuck in the tube as an ectopic pregnancy. It is also possible that the test could interfere with the implantation of an early pregnancy and so lead to a miscarriage. If the test can only be carried out during the luteal phase, then it is best to make sure that you cannot get pregnant in that cycle by either using barrier contraception or abstaining.

There are several factors that would prevent a tubal patency test from being carried out:

- If it was thought that there was a possibility that you might already be pregnant because you were late with your period.
- If you had a period at the time of the planned test — pushing blood and endometrial cells from the uterus up into the tubes could lead to later problems such as endometriosis.
- If there were symptoms such as a high temperature associated with lower abdominal pain and vaginal discharge suggesting an

acute flare-up of pelvic inflammatory disease, because the test itself could make matters very much worse and even lead to peritonitis.

- If you had 'flu and a general anaesthetic was to be used for the test it would be common sense to wait until you were fully recovered.

Gas insufflation

This test which used to be called 'blowing the tubes' is the oldest and most reliable method of checking tubal patency. It is a very simple test to carry out and a general anaesthetic is not required. Carbon dioxide gas from a special machine is 'blown' into the uterus via a cannula, an instrument gently inserted, into the cervical canal. The equipment records the pressure of the gas in the uterus; this increases initially then falls as the gas passes along the tubes. However, the problem is that it is impossible to tell whether or not the gas has passed through only one tube, both tubes or simply leaked out between the cannula and the cervical canal. Even if the test records a constant high pressure indicating that both tubes might be blocked, it will give no indication as to the site of the obstruction. Gas insufflation has, therefore, largely fallen out of use and is of historical interest mainly.

Hysterosalpingography (HSG)

A hystersalpingogram is an X-ray of the uterus and tubes. It is an out-patient procedure and is usually carried out without a general anaesthetic in the X-ray department. An instrument is gently intro-duced into the cervical canal and a radio-opaque dye (one that will show up on an X-ray) is injected slowly through it into the uterus. You may find that this causes you to experience some discomfort, rather like a period pain. As the test is being carried out, the doctor can see what is happening on an X-ray screen. If everything is normal, the uterus can be seen to fill with dye which then passes along each tube to enter the peritoneal cavity of the abdomen. If the dye is unable to enter one or both tubes it may indicate an obstruction at the junction of the uterus and tubes or simply a temporary spasm at this site. If either tube is blocked at the outer fimbrial end, the tube will become distended and will be easily seen on the screen as a **hydrosalpinx**.

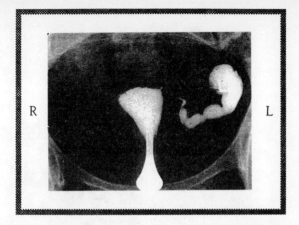

Fig. 14: Hysterosalpingogram showing a large left hydrosalpinx and no filling of the right tube which is occluded at the utero-tubal junction.

The HSG is the best method of assessing the actual shape of the cavity of the uterus. Sometimes abnormalities in the development of the uterus, which might otherwise be missed, can be picked up — a wall or septum dividing the uterine cavity, for example. The cavity of the uterus may appear to be irregular in outline or there may be what is known as a filling defect due to the presence of fibroids.

A 'normal' HSG, however, does not in itself necessarily mean that all is well. Adhesions inside the uterus can be missed on X-ray and can only be detected by using a special instrument called a hysteroscope which allows the cavity of the uterus to be inspected. Although the dye might pass freely through both tubes, this does not mean that the rest of the pelvis will get a clean bill of health. The ovaries may be enveloped in fine adhesions and there would be nothing to suggest this unless one of the tubes appeared to be hitched up or in a distorted position. Such adhesions would prevent the egg from having access to the tube.

The HSG is not always easy to interpret. It can be even more difficult if the doctor has only the X-ray films to go on and was not present at the time the X-rays were taken. If the X-ray findings alone were used to diagnose a tubal problem, then quite a significant number of women would find themselves undergoing unnecessary surgery on the basis of a misdiagnosed test: for example, tubal spasm at the junction of the tubes and uterus being mistaken for tubal obstruction. If a hysterosalpingogram only has been performed and there is some

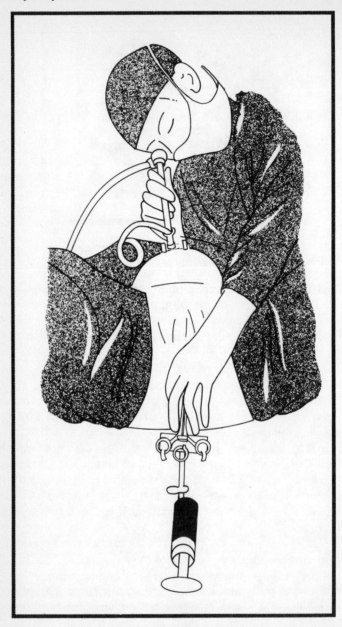

Fig. 15: Use of a laparoscope to view the pelvic cavity and check whether both tubes are open (patent).

doubt over the normality of the pelvis, then the back-up of laparoscopy is essential.

Laparoscopy

In the late 1960s, laparoscopy was popularized by Patrick Steptoe, one of the great gynaecologists of the twentieth century. It is now generally regarded as being the method of choice for tubal patency testing. It is a much more complex technique than HSG and requires admission to hospital and usually a general anaesthetic. A tiny incision is made within the lower edge of the umbilicus (where any scar will be totally invisible later). Through this incision, the abdominal cavity is distended with carbon dioxide gas. This creates a large gas-filled space which allows for much easier viewing of the pelvic organs. A slim-line telescope called a laparoscope is then introduced into the abdominal cavity, and the uterus, tubes, ovaries and neighbouring organs are thoroughly inspected (Fig. 15). The normality of the pelvis is assessed and the presence of any abnormality such as endometriosis, adhesions from pelvic inflammatory disease, and fibroids is made a note of. In the normal pelvis, the uterus, tubes and ovaries are gleaming

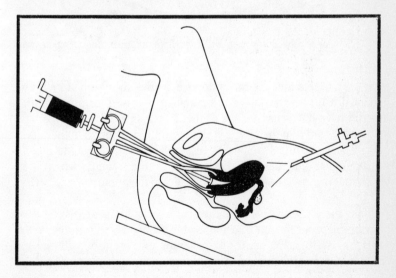

Fig. 16: To check whether both tubes are open, a harmless blue dye is syringed into the uterus.

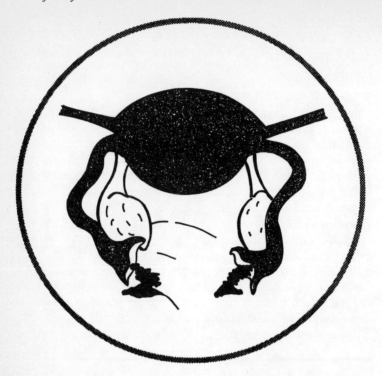

Fig. 17: View of pelvis through laparoscope. Both fallopian tubes are patent to dye.

with health. Neither the tubes nor the ovaries should in any way be stuck down by adhesions so that any egg released from the ovaries would have free access to the tubes. To assess tubal patency, a blue dye is injected into the uterus via an instrument inserted in the cervix (Fig. 16). If the tubes are patent, they will be seen to become slightly distended as they fill with dye coming from the uterus which then spills out through the fimbrial ends and into the peritoneal cavity (Fig. 17).

If the tubes are obstructed at their insertion into the uterus, no tubal filling will occur in spite of considerable pressure being applied to the injecting syringe. If a hydrosalpinx is present, the tube will be seen to become grossly distended with blue dye which does not escape from the fimbrial end. (Sometimes the dye is forced out through the sealed off fimbrial end of the tube but this nearly always closes itself off to become obstructed again.)

In addition to assessing tubal patency, fine adhesions can sometimes be divided by inserting special cauterizing scissors. Small areas of endometriosis can also be destroyed by a form of cautery known as diathermy.

After these tests, the majority of patients are able to leave hospital by the following day at the latest.

There can be no doubt that laparoscopic assessment of the pelvis has great advantages over HSG: it allows the surgeon to have a direct view of the pelvic organs and gives a much more accurate assessment of tubal patency. The need for further surgery can be simply determined at the time of laparoscopy without requiring an 'exploratory operation' which might turn out to be unnecessary.

Laparoscopy and HSG do complement each other, however. If during laparoscopy the pelvis appears to be 100 per cent normal but no dye can be seen to enter the tubes, the diagnosis could be either tubal spasm or tubal obstruction. If a subsequent HSG shows free spill of dye from each tube than it can be safely assumed that tubal spasm was responsible for the failed laparoscopic patency test.

These tests complete the basic Infertility Clinic investigations. It may be that you will both have passed all the tests with flying colours and your infertility will be labelled as 'unexplained'. It would be a mistake to be disappointed if no problem can be found at this stage because it is usually possible that further attempts at becoming pregnant will eventually succeed. This does of course depend on *all* the basic tests being carried out. Sadly, Infertility Clinics all too frequently see patients who have been told that there is no fertility problem, but when they go into the past investigations, they find that this assessment has been made on the basis of inadequate information. Post-coital tests are often left out. It is such an important test because a normal semen analysis and a good result from a correctly timed post-coital test means that your partner may be regarded as being normal. It also rules out any immunological (antibody) cause for your infertility. The spotlight instead can turn onto you! A single progesterone assay will only give information about one cycle but in order to assess the length of the luteal phase, a BBT chart at least is required. An alternative would be to carry out several progesterone assays in the cycle but this is often impractical. There are newer methods of assessing progesterone by measuring levels of the hormone in saliva. The patient simply takes all of the daily saliva samples into the laboratory at the end of a cycle. Unfortunately, this relatively simple assay is not readily available. If the luteal phase is inadequate it is usually because of poor stimulation of the ovary during the follicular phase of the cycle. This can in turn be monitored by serial hormone assays of oestrogen, progesterone, FSH and LH during the follicular phase combined with ultrasound scanning of follicular development. Ultrasound can show up defective follicular growth and also the problem of the follicle that fails to ovulate, the so-called '**luteinized unruptured follicle**' syndrome (or LUF).

If all investigations are normal and a pregnancy still does not occur, the likelihood is that there is some undetected problem with sperm movement or the sperm's ability to fertilize the egg. There are other more sophisticated tests that are available in some centres that can go some way in checking these important sperm functions. There are, for example, special photo-microscopic techniques for the examination and assessment of sperm movement. It is also known that the normal human sperm is able to fertilize a specially treated hamster egg (without producing any science fiction monster!), and it is often assumed that if this test is normal, that the sperm will also be able to fertilize the human egg. However, in-vitro fertilization ('test-tube' pregnancy) programmes have shown that this is not always the case. Some sperm are simply unable to penetrate the zona pellucida around the human egg.

The possible courses of action open to you if you have been diagnosed as having 'unexplained infertility' will be discussed in Chapter nine.

Apart from 'unexplained infertility', the basic tests are likely to have shown up a problem that is the probable cause of your infertility. The treatment of such problems will be dealt with in the following chapters.

6

Should I be on a fertility drug?

If all your tests have shown that ovulation is occurring normally, there is little point in taking a 'fertility drug' in the hope that it might somehow make a difference and 'do something' miraculous. Many gynaecologists will admit to giving such drugs on the basis that they are unlikely to do harm and may somehow do the trick. But this is really rather like taking headache tablets when you don't have a headache. The only valid reason to prescribe a fertility drug is to improve a situation that is not perfect and thereby increase the chances of a pregnancy occurring.

In Chapter one the complex interaction between the brain, pituitary gland and ovaries was described, yet even this quite detailed description was very simplified. When the whole control of ovulation is so complicated, it is easy to appreciate that it can sometimes go wrong. In at least 20 per cent of the couples attending an Infertility Clinic, there will be some defect in ovulation. Clues to a probable ovulation problem may very well come from the initial history taken at your first visit to the clinic.

If you have never had a period, a condition known as **primary amenorrhoea**, it is hardly surprising that a pregnancy has not occurred as you have not yet had a cycle in which to ovulate and produce an egg. (Incidentally, 1 per cent of normal women only have their very first period at the age of 20.)

You may on the other hand have a condition called **secondary amenorrhoea**, where periods which were once regular, have now stopped altogether.

If you are having only two or three periods a year (oligomenorrhoea), then you will have only two or three chances each year to become pregnant, instead of the 13 chances you would have with a normal four-week cycle. When ovulation does occur in these circumstances, it may be completely normal, although obviously very unpredictable. In fact, most Infertility Clinics have had the experience of a patient presenting herself with just this sort of menstrual history, and on examination, to her amazement, embarrassment, and eventual delight, an abdominal swelling is found which proves on ultrasound to be a pregnancy! Even if your oligomenorrhoea is much less severe — e.g. with periods occurring every six to eight weeks — this very unpredictability of your cycle may cause infertility.

Although the menstrual history may give the initial clue to the actual cause of your infertility, it is possible to have defective ovulation with a completely normal and regular cycle. It will only be by a combination of investigations including BBT charts, hormone profiles, progesterone assays and ultrasound, that the true problem with ovulation can be identified.

These basic investigations can reveal a number of different problems:

Polycystic ovary disease (PCOD)

This very common disorder of ovulation accounts for up to 60 per cent of ovulation problems. The cycle is usually prolonged, with oligomenorrhoea a common feature. Women who have this condition are often (although not invariably) overweight. If you have PCOD, you will be producing a little bit too much of the male hormone, testosterone. This does not mean that you are about to change your sex and turn into a man! The normal woman produces mainly oestrogen and a little testosterone, while in the man it is the other way around. As explained earlier, in PCOD, this mild overproduction of testosterone leads to a hormone imbalance, with too much LH and too little FSH being produced in the early part of the cycle. The ovaries become packed full of little follicle cysts which can be seen on both ultrasound and at laparoscopy. The follicle is unable to develop in the normal way and ovulation cannot occur.

The treatment of this condition is to reverse the topsy-turvy levels of LH and FSH, by either stimulating the pituitary to produce more FSH and to restore the balance to normal, or to achieve the same result by actually administering FSH.

Inadequate luteal phase

You will recall that the luteal phase is the second half of the cycle following ovulation, where the main feature is the production of progesterone from the corpus luteum. An inadequate luteal phase (sometimes called a 'poor', 'short' or 'insufficient' luteal phase) is often seen on BBT charts where the temperature rise after apparent ovulation lasts for less than 11 days and where correctly timed progesterone assays are less than 30 nmol per litre.

The problem, however, does not lie with the corpus luteum itself but with what was going on earlier in the cycle. The growth of an egg follicle and its subsequent release at ovulation depends upon the adequate production of FSH from the pituitary. If the FSH output is poor, receptor sites on the growing egg follicle will not be adequately prepared and primed to recognize and respond to the rise in LH, an event which leads to normal ovulation. Egg production in that cycle is likely to be poorly stimulated and even if ovulation does occur, the corpus luteum will be unable to produce the normal levels of progesterone.

The treatment required for this commonly occurring problem is to improve the stimulation of the follicle by boosting the level of FSH in the first part of the cycle. This will prime the LH receptor sites on the follicle so that ovulation will occur normally and this in turn will be followed by a normal output of progesterone from the corpus luteum.

Pituitary failure

In this situation, the pituitary gland is unable to produce FSH and LH adequately. As a result, there is no stimulation of the ovary and no egg production, leading to amenorrhoea, absence of a period. Not surprisingly, FSH, LH and oestrogen levels are extremely low.

Treatment here involves administering FSH and LH; it is usually impossible to stimulate the pituitary to produce more of these hormones by itself.

Reduced function of hypothalamus and pituitary

The hypothalamus is the area immediately above the pituitary gland

and in fact controls pituitary function. It is not uncommon for the pituitary gland and ovary to go into a prolonged 'limbo state' where the normal stimulation by the pituitary gland and response by the ovary does not occur. This is common in the months immediately after stopping the contraceptive Pill. When the Pill is being taken, there is enough oestrogen 'feedback' from the Pill to satisfy the hypothalamus. This means that the hypothalamus in turn does not stimulate the pituitary and as a result the ovaries do not receive any instructions to produce their own oestrogen. Ovulation, therefore, does not occur, which is after all the whole idea of taking the Pill in the first place. When the Pill is stopped in order to start a family, the hypothalamus, pituitary and ovaries have become so used to not having to produce hormones, that they can continue in this state of inactivity for several months. In the majority of women, the cycle does eventually return to normal, but very occasionally it can take many months to do so. This absence of periods is called **post-Pill-related amenorrhoea**. The FSH, LH and oestrogen levels are usually normal. If you have stopped the Pill because you wish to start a family and periods do not come back of their own accord, it is pointless to go on waiting, getting more and more impatient and frustrated with the whole situation. If your periods show no signs of returning within six months of stopping the Pill, there is little point in delaying further and you should get referred to a clinic earlier rather than later.

The same situation can also occur without the Pill being involved. Periods can stop altogether when there has been a dramatic loss in weight (**weight-loss-related amenorrhoea**); this can occur when drastic dieting takes place, or in serious conditions such as anorexia nervosa. Major stress states can also stop periods completely. The hypothalamus which controls the pituitary gland in turn operates under the influence of higher centres in the brain, so it is not really surprising to find that amenorrhoea can occur following major long-term emotional stress. Interestingly, the majority of first class women athletes, at the peak of physical fitness and training, will have amenorrhoea. They can voluntarily bring their periods back by training less vigorously! Their amenorrhoea is really a result of striving for perfection and is due to a combination of the loss of body fat and stress.

The treatment of post-Pill-related amenorrhoea is to break the 'limbo state' and stimulate additional pituitary FSH production. Fertility drugs are not required for weight-loss-related amenorrhoea, and indeed do not work well. The treatment here is to gain weight.

Ovarian failure

In this situation, the ovaries fail to respond to FSH from the pituitary. The commonest reason for this is that the ovaries have simply run out of eggs. This in fact represents the menopause (change of life). When this happens prematurely to a woman in her thirties who does not yet have a family the result is obviously going to be devastating. Such women all have secondary amenorrhoea; they have unmeasurably high FSH and LH levels and rock-bottom oestrogen levels. A pregnancy is going to be impossible other than by egg donation from another woman.

Very rarely, the ovaries are resistant to FSH and LH and are unable to respond. Treatment of this condition is complicated and involves suppressing the pituitary gland for a period and then artificially stimulating the ovaries with FSH.

Hyperprolactinaemia

In this quite common condition, there is an excessive production of the pituitary hormone, prolactin. This is the hormone normally responsible for milk production after having a baby. Sometimes the normal pituitary simply produces too much of this hormone, but occasionally a tiny benign (non-malignant) tumour of the pituitary called a prolactinoma is the cause of the high prolactin. This interferes with the production of FSH and LH and oligomenorrhoea or secondary amenorrhoea results.

After additional investigations, treatment involves using drugs to lower the high prolactin level and so allow for the normal production of FSH and LH.

Fertility drug treatment

Apart from ovarian failure, all of the above disorders of ovulation can be corrected with fertility drugs. It is not necessary to have completed all of your investigations before starting treatment, except in the case of the most complex (and expensive) treatment programmes. If, say, you have oligomenorrhoea, and there are no other obvious problems suggested by your history and examination and preliminary tests, it would be perfectly reasonable to start off treatment as soon as your immunity to Rubella has been confirmed. The patency of your tubes could at least initially be given the benefit of the doubt as the particular treatment involved in treating this condition is relatively straightforward and the drugs used are reasonably cheap.

A preliminary test that often precedes drug treatment proper, is based on an understanding of the normal menstrual cycle. During the normal cycle, oestrogen production by the follicle, and then progesterone production from the corpus luteum, renew the lining endometrium of the uterus shed with the last period. If a pregnancy does not occur, the progesterone level falls and a period follows shortly afterwards. However, the period will only occur after the progesterone fall if the endometrium has first been primed and prepared by the normal production of oestrogen during the first half of the cycle. This natural sequence of events forms the basis of the test.

If you have amenorrhoea, your oestrogen levels can be assessed by giving you a five-day course of progesterone tablets. If you are producing small amounts of oestrogen, as in pituitary failure, nothing will happen after stopping the course of progesterone. You will get no withdrawal bleed because the endometrium will not have been primed by oestrogen. If, on the other hand, you have post-Pill related amenorrhoea, your oestrogen levels will be normal, the pituitary and ovaries having only been lulled to sleep by their months of inactivity while you have been on the Pill. The normal levels of oestrogen will have had a priming effect on the endometrium, so that shortly after finishing the five days on progesterone, a withdrawal bleed occurs.

The practical value of this **'progesterone challenge' test** is that certain fertility drugs require the levels of oestrogen to be normal in order to bring about ovulation. If your oestrogen levels are low to start with, these particular fertility drugs will have no effect. The progesterone challenge test therefore identifies which of the patients with amenorrhoea are likely to respond to a particular treatment.

A variety of fertility drugs are used to stimulate ovulation. The principal drugs, all of which I will discuss, are clomiphene, cyclofenil, human chorionic gonadotrophin (HGC), bromocriptine, human menopausal gonadotrophin (HMG), urofollitrophin (pure FSH), gonadotrophin releasing hormone (GnRH or LHRH).

Clomiphene

Clomiphene is a commonly used fertility drug. It is very effective in correcting defective ovulation when the levels of oestrogen in the body are normal. In such women, the progesterone challenge test would be positive in that they would have a withdrawal bleed after stopping the five-day course of progesterone tablets. Clomiphene, therefore, is essentially an anti-oestrogen drug because it interrupts the feedback of oestrogen to the hypothalamus. By blocking the normal oestrogen receptors on the hypothalamus, clomiphene is really fooling the brain into thinking that there is an inadequate level of circulating oestrogen. By giving the hypothalamus a nudge, this 'wakes up' the whole system and the rest works by 'knock-on' effect leading eventually to ovulation.

Climophene treatment is beneficial in the following situations:

- If you have amenorrhoea (e.g. post-Pill) and a positive progesterone challenge test.
- If you have oligomenorrhoea with periods that are few and far between (this includes polycystic ovary disease, PCOD).
- If your BBT chart and/or your day 21 progesterone assays suggest inadequate luteal phases.
- If you are to receive donor insemination (DI) it is important that ovulation is as regular and as predictable as possible.

Treatment with clomiphene is very safe. It is not a drug that will make you have five or six babies at once, but twins are certainly commoner, being in the region of 1 in 16 pregnancies (approximately six per cent), instead of the 1 in 80 chance for the general population.

Before starting you on treatment with clomiphene, you will be made aware of the possible side-effects. If these do occur they are very mild, and it is rare that treatment has to stop because of them. The commonest side effect is hot flushes, which occur in about 10 per cent of patients. It is due to the anti-oestrogen effect of the tablets and not to the change of life! Occasional headaches may occur, but you can take whatever pain relieving medication you would normally use and this will not clash with the clomiphene. Some women feel depressed while taking clomiphene, but a lot of women feel like this during a period anyway. In addition, if you have had a good response to the clomiphene and a period arrives, you are going to feel a bit down in the dumps that it didn't work that cycle. One quite unusual side-effect can affect your vision: when you come out of the dark into a brightly lit room, coloured objects can almost flash their colours at you and your vision can become blurred until your eyes get used to the light. Very occasionally breast discomfort, abdominal distension, and slight weight gain may occur. The only symptom which might mean that you should have a short break from treatment would be the development of pelvic pain. This quite rare problem is due to temporary enlargement of the ovaries and is a mild form of over-stimulation.

Treatment starts within the first five days of your period beginning, whether this period was a natural period or a withdrawal bleed from a progesterone challenge test. Depending upon your specialist, the initial dosage of clomiphene will vary from 1 tablet (50 mg) to 2 tablets (100 mg) daily for 4-5 days. Ovulation will normally occur 5-13 days after the last clomiphene tablet. While on this treatment, I feel it is of value for you to keep a BBT chart, so that both you and the clinic can keep a check on the occurrence and timing of ovulation. Day 21 progesterone assays will also usually be carried out to confirm the probability of ovulation. Some clinics are able to offer ultrasound tracking of the follicle's growth.

If your response to clomiphene is considered to be inadequate, the dosage can be increased by 1-2 tablets per day to a maximum dose of 4 tablets (200 mg) daily. The majority of patients will ovulate at the 100 mg per day dosage level. Once ovulation has been shown to occur at a particular level, there is no point in increasing the dosage further. Treatment is usually maintained at this dosage for six cycles and examples, taken from actual BBT charts, are shown below.

Case 1

The chart below belongs to a patient with post-Pill-related amenorrhoea. She had a positive progesterone challenge test after 5 days of progesterone (P) tablets taken twice daily. She then commenced clomiphene (C) tablets 50 mg twice daily which she took for 4 days. It can be seen from the fall and rise of temperature that she ovulated on day 23 of the cycle, 10 days after the last clomiphene tablet. The equivalent of a day 21 progesterone assay

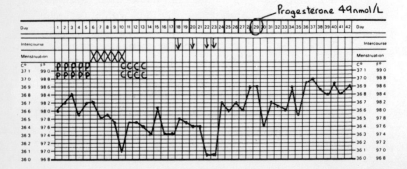

confirmed ovulation. The temperature remained elevated and a pregnancy was confirmed.

Case 2

This patient had oligomenorrhoea with a 6-8 week cycle associated with polycystic ovary disease. In the first chart there is no evidence of ovulation at all; the temperature simply zig-zags along the bottom of the chart for nearly 9 weeks, going onto a second chart before a period commenced. (The chart shows the 6 weeks leading up to that period.)

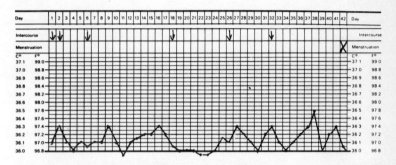

Clomiphene 100 mg daily was then given for 4 days commencing on the second day of the period. The clomiphene has stimulated the release of FSH from the pituitary restoring the normal balance between LH and FSH. Ovulation occurred on day 14 and the patient became pregnant after her first course of treatment.

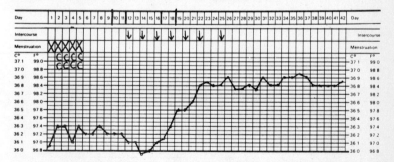

Case 3

The first two BBT charts below show grossly inadequate luteal phases. Day 21 progesterone assays were very low.

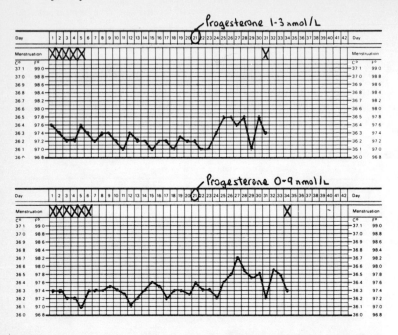

This patient then received clomiphene 100 mg daily for 4 days. In her first course of treatment the luteal phase improved considerably when an improved progesterone output, and in the second course she became pregnant. (On the second course, day 21 occurred before a delayed ovulation. If a BBT chart had not been kept, it could easily have been initially assumed that she had not ovulated at all! Another advantage of the BBT chart is that when a pregnancy does occur it pinpoints the date of conception and the expected date of delivery with greater accuracy than even ultrasound.)

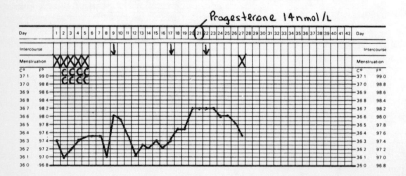

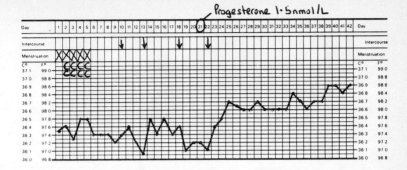

Case 4

This patient who has a 30-40-day cycle is ovulating well with good luteal phases and good day 21 progesterones. However, she is having problems in timing her attendances for donor insemination. She has a moderately irregular cycle·and therefore unpredictable ovulation.

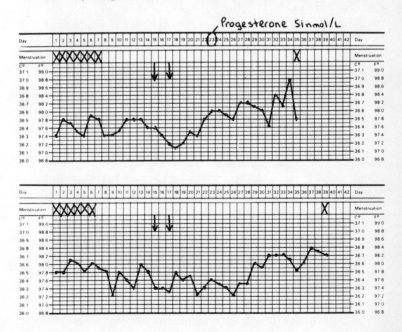

This patient started clomiphene 100 mg daily for 4 days which rapidly made ovulation predictable and she became pregnant after her second cycle of treatment.

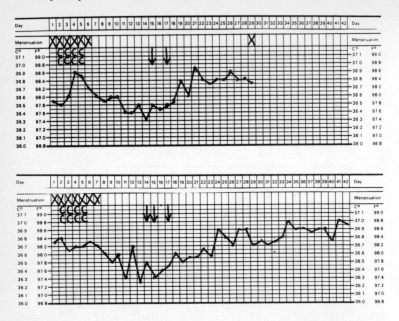

If a correctly timed post-coital test was negative before starting treatment with clomiphene, it may have been due to the fact that you were not growing an egg follicle normally and not producing sufficient oestrogen to stimulate mucus secretion by the glands of the cervix. Once ovulation has been adequately stimulated in cycles on clomiphene, there is usually (but not always) a dramatic improvement in cervical mucus secretion. Furthermore, ovulation timing is made more predictable and it is easier to time your post-coital test for the correct day of the cycle. It is *most important* to have your post-coital test repeated if it was poor or negative before commencing clomiphene treatment.

You will recall that I have several times commented on the anti-oestrogen action of clomiphene. This means that clomiphene will cause the release of FSH and actually increase subsequent oestrogen production while maturing an egg follicle. Although clomiphene can stimulate normal ovulation, sometimes its anti-oestrogen activity can have a lasting effect on the cervical mucus. Instead of being flowing and watery, the mucus can become scanty and almost glue-like and no normal sperm movement can be seen within it. For this reason, even if your post-coital test was perfect before going onto clomiphene, the test should be repeated once you are on treatment to make sure that the mucus remains satisfactory.

If the post-coital test shows this unwanted side effect of clomiphene, a pregnancy is unlikely to occur unless this hostile factor can be removed. Indeed, very unfavourable mucus can almost act like a contraceptive! Reducing the dosage of clomiphene may occasionally be of benefit to the mucus but the price may be an inadequate luteal phase. I have found that the addition of a natural oestrogen after the clomiphene can often counteract this unwanted aspect of its anti-oestrogen effect and restore the mucus to normal.

Case 5

This patient was receiving clomiphene which corrected inadequate luteal phases. At post-coital testing on day 14 of the cycle, the mucus was thick and virtually non-existent. No sperm were seen within it.

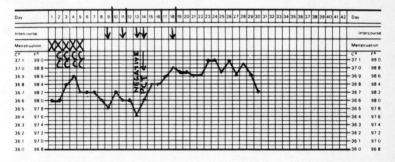

As a result, she was given oestrogen (O) after the clomiphene. You will see that the oestrogen tablets were given in a rising dosage to mimic the normal oestrogen rise that occurs before ovulation (Fig. 8). The post-coital test on day 15 showed superb mucus with an active sperm population. As a bonus she got pregnant as well!

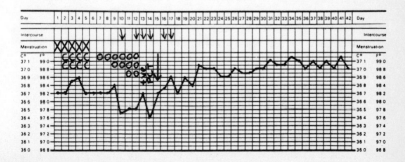

I have found that the addition of oestrogen is usually helpful when the mucus is unfavourable on clomiphene. However, it does seem a little odd to be giving one particular treatment to correct one problem and then have to use another drug to correct the side effects of the first treatment. Some centres are going back to the use of a drug that has been available for many years, **cyclofenil**. It is similar to clomiphene in its action and it is said to have less in the way of side effects. A reported advantage of cyclofenil is that the cervical mucus remains watery and flowing. The dosage is 2 100 mg tablets daily for 10 days commencing on day 3 of the period. Personally, I have not found it to be as good as clomiphene at stimulating ovulation.

Sometimes the luteal phase remains short in spite of what seems to be adequate stimulation with clomiphene. Day 21 progesterone levels are normal but the length of the luteal phase is less than the 11 days required to allow for normal implantation of a fertilized egg. In such cases, it can be very beneficial to stimulate the corpus luteum more vigorously so that there is a more prolonged output of progesterone. This luteal phase support extends the length of the luteal phase and increases the chance of implantation.

Enhancing implantation can be accomplished by administering a hormone normally made by the early embryo and placenta, **human chorionic gonadotrophin** or **HCG**. This hormone is identical in its action to LH. If it is given at the time of the expected LH surge (Figs. 7 & 8), an egg that has been sufficiently matured by clomiphene will then ovulate. The HCG is given by an intramuscular injection of 5,000 units (1 ampoule) to 10,000 units. If the luteal phase is still inadequate, a second injection of 5,000 units a week later may promote further progesterone output from the corpus luteum and so give sufficient time for a fertilized egg to implant. But be warned! This second injection can be a bit hard on your nerves as sometimes the extended length of the luteal phase can mistakenly raise false hopes.

Case 6

This patient was given clomiphene for irregular cycles with inadequate luteal phases. It can be seen that although ovulation has occurred more predictably, the luteal phases are still too short. The day 21 progesterone assays, however, are normal.

In the next cycle, HCG 5,000 units was given on day 13 of the cycle. The luteal phase improvement was dramatic.

On clomiphene, normal ovulation can be produced in 80-90 per cent of patients. The pregnancy rate, however, is not so high, being

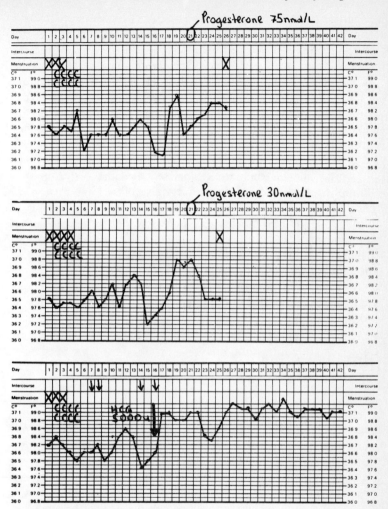

approximately 55 per cent. The reason for this difference between ovulation and pregnancy rates is that quite a number of couples will have more than one factor contributing to their infertility. If an ovulation defect is the only problem, and you fall into one of the categories suitable for treatment with clomiphene, then you can expect a pregnancy rate almost as high as the ovulation rate.

I have already stated that treatment with clomiphene is safe. It is difficult to seriously over-stimulate the ovaries using normal dosages. No treatment in medicine can guarantee a perfect end result, but I have found that the miscarriage rate among clomiphene pregnancies is at nine per cent and is therefore significantly lower than for the general population where miscarriages occur between 15-25 per cent of pregnancies conceived. One reason for this may be that clomiphene will stimulate the growth and maturation of a 'better egg'. Another factor may be that the improved FSH production after clomiphene stimulation develops sufficient LH receptors on the follicle, so that ovulation occurs normally and the corpus luteum functions in an ideal manner.

For women who have unexplained recurrent miscarriages, it might be worthwhile for them to deliberately become pregnant on a clomiphene cycle and thus to take advantage of the lower miscarriage rate. Strictly speaking, such women are not infertile, but a clomiphene-induced pregnancy may have a better chance of continuing successfully.

Babies resulting from clomiphene treatment do not have an increased chance of abnormality.

In recent years some specialists have been using another anti-oestrogen drug called **tamoxifen**, which is very similar to clomiphene.

Bromocriptine

Prolactin is the pituitary hormone responsible for milk production (lactation) after the delivery of a baby. Sometimes there can be an excessive production of prolactin in a woman who has not recently been pregnant. The high levels of prolactin interfere with the normal signal from the hypothalamus to the pituitary, so that there is a reduction in FSH and LH output. As a result, oligomenorrhoea and even amenorrhoea may occur. About one-third of the women who have this condition of hyperprolactinaemia will actually be producing milk. This inappropriate lactation is known as **galactorrhoea**. In a way, this mimics what normally happens during breast feeding, where the return of periods may be delayed until the baby has been weaned.

Measurement of your prolactin levels should be routine if you have any menstrual irregularity. The level of prolactin is held to be significantly raised, if it is at least double the upper limit of the normal 450 mU/L. Repeat testing should be used to confirm high prolactin levels. All sorts of things can push your prolactin level up. The stress of even having a blood test can have an immediate effect on prolactin levels, especially if you have to wait in a long queue for your test, getting increasingly apprehensive as you move closer to the pin prick! However, the rise in prolactin from stress is not too drastic and repeat tests are usually found to be normal. Certain drugs including some of the tranquillizers and blood pressure lowering drugs can be associated with raised prolactin levels. In some women, the pituitary gland will simply over-produce prolactin without any obvious cause being found. The most important cause is the development of a microscopic benign (non malignant) tumour of the pituitary gland called a **prolactinoma**. The area of the skull that houses the pituitary gland is called the pituitary fossa (Fig. 4), and this is easy to investigate. A simple skull X-ray will not reveal very much, but sophisticated X-rays (known as coned lateral tomography) will show if there has been any enlargement of the pituitary fossa which would indicate a probable prolactinoma. Even better measurement of the pituitary gland itself can be obtained using special scans known as CAT or CT (computed tomography) scans. The remarkable thing about the majority of prolactinomas is that they can be made to virtually disappear within a few days using a fertility drug called bromocriptine. This drug is the treatment of choice for hyperprolactinaemia whether or not a prolactinoma is present. It is very rare to have to consider surgical treatment for a prolactinoma, surgery only being indicated for very large tumours that cannot be shrunk down in size.

Bromocriptine rapidly lowers prolactin levels so that there is no longer any suppression of the hypothalamus. FSH production recommences with a return of ovulation and a normal cycle. It is, however, essential that the tablets are always taken with food so as to avoid severe nausea, vomiting and diarrhoea. Other side effects that may occasionally occur are headaches, dizziness, and general lassitude. Usually the clinic will advise you to start off on half of a 2.5 mg tablet a day with food and slowly build up to a maintenance dose of 2-3 tablets (5-7.5 mg) per day. It is important to remeasure the prolactin level once your treatment has been established. If treatment is effective, the prolactin levels should be pushed down well below the upper limit of normal. If you were originally found to have a large prolactinoma, scanning of the pituitary gland will be repeated while you are on treatment to make sure that the pituitary has returned to normal size. The bromocriptine tablets are continued daily, often with BBT chart control unit there is evidence of a pregnancy, when the treatment is stopped. Some patients will require the addition of clomiphene to their bromocriptine therapy if ovulation is not satisfactory.

If there are no other infertility factors apart from hyper-prolactinaemia, the pregnancy rate on treatment with bromocriptine is in the region of 80 per cent. These pregnancies do not have an increased miscarriage rate and the treatment has not been shown to cause any problem to the unborn baby.

A prolactinoma that was present before pregnancy will not cause any problems during pregnancy itself unless it was excessively large to start with and had not shrunk down with treatment. I must stress that this is an exceedingly rare complication.

Human menopausal gonadotrophin (HMG)

If you have developed amenorrhoea, you will be thoroughly investigated before any treatment starts in order to determine the cause of the amenorrhoea. This not only makes sound medical sense but also justifies the considerable expense of some of the treatments. For example, it would be absurd to treat you with very powerful fertility drugs if your absence of periods was due to ovarian failure because of the menopause! A full hormone profile will therefore exclude this and other causes of amenorrhoea such as hyper-prolactinaemia. Similarly, your partner's semen analysis must be normal and your tubal patency must be confirmed by laparoscopy before you start on complex treatment. It would after all be ridiculous to embark on such treatment and subsequently find that the sperm count was unsatisfactory or that your tubes were blocked.

If your pituitary gland fails to produce FSH and LH, your ovaries will in turn fail to mature eggs. Oestrogen production by the ovaries will be very low, ovulation will not occur and amenorrhoea will result. As a result of the inadequate production of oestrogen, the endometrium of the uterus will not be primed and a progesterone challenge test will be negative. This means that there will not be a withdrawal bleed after five days of progesterone tablets.

The only way in which you are likely to become pregnant is if you are given the FSH and LH that the pituitary gland is failing to make for itself. It may surprise you that the source of the FSH and LH used for such treatment is the urine of post-menopausal women. (After the menopause the ovaries stop producing oestrogen and in response to this the levels of FSH and LH are very high. These raised levels of hormones are excreted into the urine.) The FSH and LH are extracted from the urine and purified. Each resulting ampoule of HMG contains 75 international units (IU) of both FSH and LH.

Treatment with HMG is complex. I generally find that it takes me an hour to adequately counsel a couple about HMG and explain the intricacies of treatment to them. It is essential that the consequences of treatment with HMG are thoroughly appreciated.

HMG is the drug that sometimes makes the headlines when a woman has three or more babies. Out of my first 100 pregnancies on HMG, 70 per cent were single pregnancies, 25 per cent were twins and 5 per cent were triplets. In other words, 95 per cent of the pregnancies occurring after treatment with HMG resulted in one or two babies.

If you are given HMG, your ovaries will respond to the FSH in the preparation and egg maturation will take place. As a result, your oestrogen levels will rise and this provides a very handy method of assessing your response to treatment. The oestrogen can be easily measured by 24-hour urine collections which will indicate whether your response to HMG has been poor, fair, good, very good or excessive. The aim of treatment is to produce oestrogen levels between 180 and 514 nmol per 24-hour urine collection. If the final oestrogen level is below 180 nmol, a pregnancy is unlikely to occur. If the level is above 514 nmol, the risks of a multiple pregnancy increase. The importance of accurate urine collections can be appreciated if this is going to be the chief method of monitoring your response to HMG. Unfortunately, the oestrogen levels in themselves do not indicate the number of follicles that are likely to ovulate. However, scanning of the ovaries with ultrasound will demonstrate the number of follicles that are growing and is a very helpful additional method of assessing the effectiveness of treatment.

There are two main ways in which treatment can be given with HMG. It can either be given by three equal injections of HMG on alternate days or by a daily injection programme. Response to treatment is assessed by 24-hour urine assays and ultrasound. The dosage is increased until a satisfactory oestrogen level is reached. Sometimes clomiphene is given with the HMG with an improvement in the results. The HMG, however, will only produce growth of the follicle. In order to bring about ovulation, HCG 10,000 units is given by injection. You will not ovulate without the HCG. It is obviously important that intercourse should take place at this time of the treatment cycle. If you do not get pregnant after a course of HMG/HCG treatment, a period will occur. If the oestrogen level is sky-high, the HCG will be withheld so as to avoid the risks of both a very multiple pregnancy and a complication known as hyperstimulation syndrome. If the HCG is not given, a period begins a few days later and treatment could be recommenced.

Hyperstimulation will only occur if the final oestrogen level before the HCG injection is high or has risen very sharply within the normal range. It cannot occur unless th HCG has been given. Mild hyperstimulation occurs in about 5 per cent of all treatment cycles and shows up as abdominal distension and pain due to enlarged ovaries. A high proportion of hyperstimulation cycles result in a pregnancy which is an acceptable reward for having to put up with some discomfort! If a pregnancy does not result, a period follows and the ovarian enlargement rapidly disappears. Severe hyperstimulation is fortunately rare. It occurs in less than half of 1 per cent of cycles.

Treatment with HMG is most effective in the patient with amenorrhoea due to pituitary failure. However, HMG can also be used in women who fail to ovulate satisfactorily on clomiphene although the results here are less successful. One characteristic feature of HMG/HCG therapy is the cascade of cervical mucus that occurs at the time of ovulation. This beneficial 'side effect' of HMG can be taken advantage of by those women who may be ovulating very well, say on clomiphene, but who have poor or non-existent mucus at post-coital testing.

Case 7

This patient with amenorrhoea had a good response to HMG on her oestrogen rise but both the luteal phase on her temperature chart and the progesterone level were poor. A period occurred.

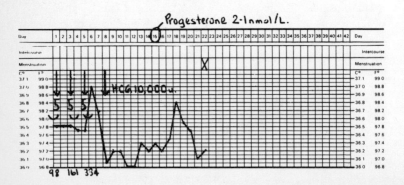

Note: (Each ↓ indicates an injection of HMG and the number of ampoules given. Each ‿ represents a 24-hour urine collection with the oestrogen level beneath it.)

In the next treatment cycle, the same HMG dosage was administered. A good 24-hour oestrogen level was obtained. One week after the HCG injection the progesterone level was very satisfactory at 132 nmol/L. A pregnancy was later confirmed and resulted in the delivery of a live, healthy, single baby.

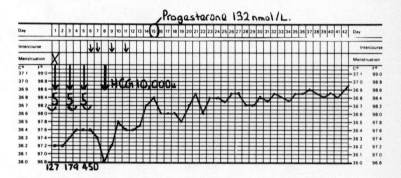

Case 8

This patient with amenorrhoea did not respond well to three alternate day treatments with HMG, as further injections were required to get an adequate oestrogen response and ovulation.

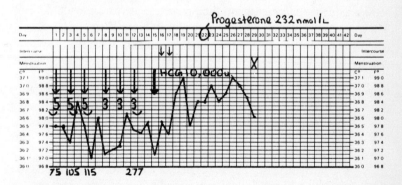

The treatment programme was changed to daily injections. On this patient's first course of daily HMG the oestrogen levels rose too high to 1140 nmol/L. The HCG was not given and a period followed.

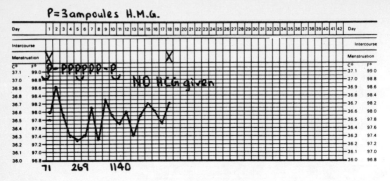

In the next cycle, the daily dosage was reduced and an excellent response was obtained with a single pregnancy.

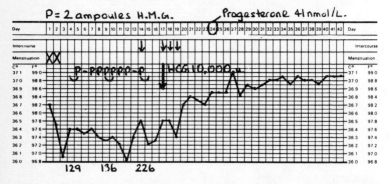

If your infertility is due solely to pituitary failure, treatment with HMG is highly successful and the pregnancy levels approach that of the normal fertile population. The majority of the pregnancies occur within six cycles of treatment. When your infertility is due to other causes, such as poor or absent ovulation and your menstrual cycle is regular, the success of HMG is reduced.

Because of the increased multiple pregnancy rates, the miscarriage rate on HMG is certainly increased. There is no increase in the abnormality rate amongst the babies delivered.

Pure FSH (Urofollitrophin)

Polycystic ovary disease (PCOD) is one of the commonest defects of ovulation. You will recall that in this condition there is an imbalance in the levels of LH and FSH, so that there is a much greater output of LH than FSH. As a result, normal growth of egg follicles does not occur. In order to rectify this situation the hormone imbalance must be corrected. The treatment options are to either stimulate the pituitary gland to increase FSH production or to actually give FSH directly.

The first line of treatment is to take advantage of the anti-oestrogen effect of clomiphene (page 85), which, by increasing pituitary FSH output certainly leads to better follicular development and ovulation. About 75 per cent of women with PCOD will ovulate on clomiphene but only one third will achieve a pregnancy. The reason for this discrepancy may be that although the FSH level has increased with clomiphene treatment, the LH levels are still high and this is thought to interfere with normal egg development.

If clomiphene should fail, the next step is to use pure FSH. The source of pure FSH is exactly the same as for HMG but the LH is withdrawn leaving only the FSH. Each ampoule contains 75 international units of pure FSH alone. The whole pre-treatment work-up is identical to that for HMG. Like HMG, the pure FSH is administered solely by injection either on alternate days or on a daily regimen. Exactly the same monitoring is required with 24-hour urine collections to measure the oestrogen response. Here too ultrasound can be very helpful. Identical precautions are taken as for HMG as similar hyperstimulation problems and multiple pregnancies can occur.

It could be argued, why not simply use HMG? While HMG will deliver the FSH, it also contains an equal amount of LH and it's the LH which causes the problem in PCOD. There is also evidence that when pure FSH is used, there is actually a reduction in the natural LH production with a pregnancy rate approaching the ovulation rate.

Case 9

Susan was 24 years old and had been married for 18 months during which time she gained 42 pounds in weight. Her periods had always been irregular and now occurred every three months.

On investigation, she had a very high LH level in contrast to a rather low FSH. Her testosterone (male hormone) level was significantly raised. Her history, the clinical findings, and the hormone results all suggested PCOD. This was confirmed at laparoscopy when the ovaries were seen to be enlarged with multiple (polycystic) grey translucent cysts within them. The tubes were patent. The semen analysis was normal. She was immune to Rubella.

She was treated first with clomiphene 100 mg daily for four days. A 45-day and 55-day cycle was produced with only debatable evidence of ovulation.

Susan was then commenced on pure FSH five ampoules on alternate days. The oestrogen levels rose to 177 nmol and she was given HCG. The luteal phase was quite good and the progesterone level was only 22 nmol/L. A period followed.

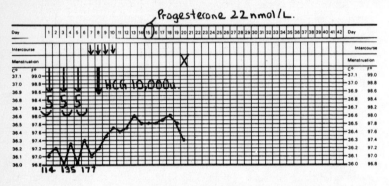

In the next course the dosage of pure FSH was increased to seven ampoules on alternate days. Although the oestrogen level was improved, the progesterone level was low. She did not ovulate.

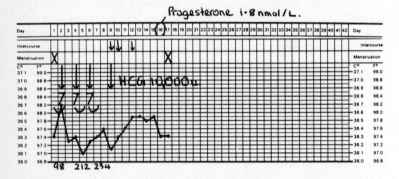

In the next cycle continuous pure FSH treatment was given on a daily basis. The oestrogen rise was very satisfactory. The progesterone level 1 week after the HCG was 43 nmol/L. A single pregnancy was confirmed shortly afterwards.

In common with HMG therapy, the majority of the pregnancies will occur within six cycles of treatment.

In some patients with PCOD, the levels of LH can be extremely high and make successful treatment with pure FSH less likely. It is sometimes worthwhile to reduce such very high LH levels before commencing treatment with pure FSH. This is called '**down**

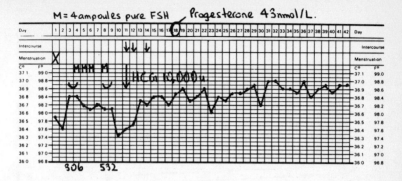

regulation' of the pituitary gland. The drug used to achieve this is called **buserelin** and prevents the pituitary gland from releasing FSH and LH. It is taken as a nasal spray several times a day and continued while on treatment with pure FSH until the day HCG is administered.

Gonadotrophin releasing hormone (GnRH or LHRH)

So far I have dealt with amenorrhoea due to a number of causes. These have included reduced function of the hypothalamus and pituitary as in post-Pill and weight-loss-related amenorrhoea, ovarian failure, hyperprolactinaemia, pituitary failure and PCOD. Another cause of amenorrhoea is hypothalamic failure.

The hypothalamus in the brain directly controls the pituitary gland. Gonadotrophin releasing hormone (GnRH) is released by the normal hypothalamus in a pulsating manner. This pulse of GnRH signals the release of FSH and LH which are stored in the pituitary. (To illustrate this, when clomiphene is taken to improve fertility, it has an anti-oestrogen effect on the hypothalamus which in fact works by increasing the frequency of these pulses of GnRH. As a result, the pituitary is stimulated to increase the output of FSH.)

Sometimes the hypothalamus fails to function normally with a defect in the GnRH pulsed release. The knock-on effect of reduced GnRH will be poor pituitary production of FSH and LH and amenorrhoea. The logical solution is to administer the missing GnRH. Synthetic GnRH has been available for several years. This, however, will only be effective if it is given in a pulsatile manner to closely mimic the normal healthy hypothalamus. It is also required to be given over a long period of time.

The delivery system to administer GnRH is a small lightweight battery-powered pump which is worn in a holster under the armpit

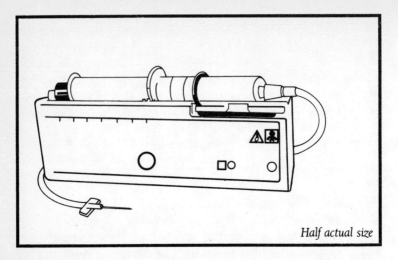

Half actual size

Fig. 18: Battery-operated pump that delivers pulsed doses of gonadatrophin releasing hormone (GnRH) through needle inserted under the skin.

day and night (Fig. 18). The pump is pre-set to deliver a 'pulse' of GnRH every 90 minutes via a small needle under the skin. This means that there will be 16 pulses every 24 hours. It is surprising how rapidly you become used to having to wear this 'robot'. My patients have devised all sorts of ingenious ways of coping with the problem of sleeping with both the pump and partner! Because there is a 90-minute breather in between pulses of treatment, it is a simple matter to detach the pump for a bath, swim or any other desired activity and get 'plugged-in' in time for the next dose. The needle requires to be resited every 48 hours. Most patients learn how to do this themselves, or if very trusting let their partners replace it. Every week you must return to the clinic to have the pump reloaded and to have a blood test to measure your FSH, LH, oestrogen and progesterone levels. The measurement of these hormones, a BBT chart, and, if available, the additional information from ultrasound scanning of the ovaries, will monitor your response to treatment. GnRH treatment is continued until pregnancy is confirmed. The vast majority of pregnancies will occur within three months of treatment. There is little point in continuing treatment for more than six months.

All this sounds very complex and cumbersome. The pumps really are very unobtrusive and are hidden by normal clothing. The big advantage that GnRH has over treatments such as HMG is that the multiple pregnancy rate is the same as for the general population with a 1 in 80 incidence of twins. Furthermore, hyperstimulation syndrome cannot occur.

The pumps are, of course, an expensive item for any clinic to stock. It is usually only major infertility centres that can offer this treatment. It is important that there is no other bar to normal fertility. If correct patient selection has been made, treatment with GnRH is highly successful, restoring fertility to normal.

The miscarriage rate is no higher than normal. The babies born do not show any increase in abnormalities.

Case 10

Jackie was 29 years of age and presented with a four year history of infertility. Her periods had been regular, occurring every 30 days, but during the previous year she had had only two periods.

On investigation she was found to be immune to Rubella and her husband's semen analysis was normal. Her hormone profile showed low normal levels of FSH, LH, oestrogen, testosterone and prolactin. There was no evidence of PCOD or hyperprolatinaemia.

At laparoscopy, the pelvis was essentially normal, although small cysts were seen in the ovaries. Both tubes were found to be patent to dye.

She had initially been treated with clomiphene, but this failed to produce ovulation. It was therefore decided to treat her with HMG. Out of six courses of treatment, she had four reasonable responses with evidence of ovulation. Unfortunately she failed to become pregnant.

It was at this time that GnRH had just become available. I decided that she would be suitable for this line of treatment. I was able to borrow a pump for the pulsed administration of the GnRH. She was

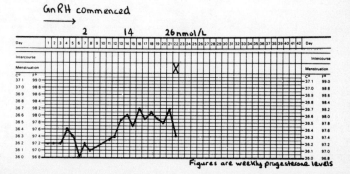

Figures are weekly progesterone levels

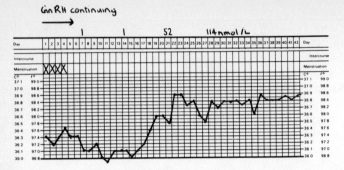

monitored with weekly hormone studies and a BBT chart (above).
Within six weeks of treatment she became pregnant. She had a
healthy son.

7

Will an operation help?

The need for some surgical procedure or another may be apparent to the specialist at your very first consultation. On the other hand, surgery may only be an option to consider if a problem is found as a result of a subsequent investigation.

I have already described the commonly performed procedure of laparoscopy. This is the ultimate diagnostic test of the normality of the fallopian tubes and also determines the general health of the pelvis. There are a number of options that may be indicated either by the initial examination in the clinic or as a result of findings revealed at laparoscopy. The decision as to whether or not to embark upon a particular operation should only be made after a full discussion of what it is hoped will be achieved by that operation, balanced against the other options that there may be to choose from. This chapter discusses the various surgical procedures that may be required to adequately treat your infertility. For the sake of simplicity, I will leave a full discussion of the options to Chapter nine.

Vaginal surgery

It is not uncommon to find that a couple's infertility is simply due to a mechanical problem in that penetration has not been occurring during intercourse. This may be due to tenderness at the vaginal entrance combined with an understandable fear of being hurt. This fear will cause the pelvic muscles to tighten and so further narrow down the vaginal entrance. Sometimes a very simple examination technique can work like magic. This is first explained to you so as to build up your confidence. Having assured you that you will not feel any pain, and that no forceful examination will be performed, you are asked to bear down strongly onto a lubricated gloved finger which is gently placed at the vaginal entrance. The bearing down movement actually relaxes the pelvic floor muscles and often to your surprise the examining finger is completely within the vagina. This can be repeated with two fingers just as easily. You can be taught to carry out this examination on yourself, so that you can practice perhaps while you are feeling relaxed in a warm bath. If you also teach your partner how to carry out this examination, your fears should dissolve away and one thing may lead to another!

Sometimes, when the history is taken, there may be no clue at all to the problem, but immediately on examination it becomes obvious that the vaginal entrance is very narrow indeed. A full vaginal examination may be impossible to perform because of an intact **hymen** (the skin fold that partially closes the entrance to the vagina in a virgin). **Vaginal dilatation** or stretching is therefore required in order to allow intercourse to take place. With patience, gentleness and care, it is usually possible to teach you how to stretch the vaginal entrance yourself. Lying on your back, a lubricated smooth, slim, blunt dilator made of toughened glass is positioned at the entrance of the vagina (Fig. 19a).

Gradual very gentle but persistent pressure is applied in an upward direction towards the back until the entire dilator is within the vagina (Fig. 19b). If this can be managed, the dilator is then held in position for a few moments, then withdrawn and gently and slowly inserted

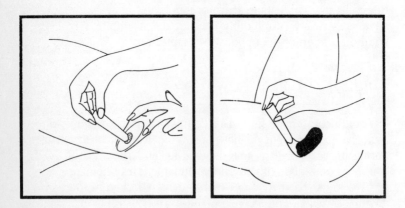

Fig. 19: To accomplish vaginal dilatation, a blunt dilator is positioned at the vaginal entrance (a) before being gently inserted (b).

again. This should be carried out 2-3 times every morning and evening until the dilator can be inserted easily without the woman experiencing any discomfort. The next size dilator is then used. If it is practical, I like to see patients return to the clinic each week to see my very capable clinic sister who checks that the dilating is progressing well. Again, it is simply a matter of building up confidence. The idea is that hopefully a time will come shortly afterwards, when your partner's 'natural' dilator can be used instead. It's worth all the effort when you return to the clinic with a big smile, saying, 'I don't need these anymore!' Usually no further treatment is required. Strictly speaking, you have never had infertility. The tight vaginal entrance preventing full intercourse was acting as a contraceptive. If there are no other obvious problems, I discharge you from the clinic telling you to 'get on with it!'

However, a significant proportion of these patients will not be able to cope with the dilators. This means that a full general anaesthetic will be required so that a thorough 'stretch up' can be performed painlessly. Occasionally it is found at that time that stretching the vaginal entrance itself is not sufficient because of a very tight ridge of skin at the lower edge of the entrance to the vagina. A simple operation known as a **perineoplasty** will correct this. This is a plastic surgery technique and consists of a small operation at the entrance to the vagina which very effectively widens the vaginal entrance. This operation can usually be performed as a day case or at the most needs an overnight stay. It is rare to need to use dilators after this operation.

There are some women who are still unable to allow penetration to take place at intercourse, regardless of the fact that there is found to be adequate room when a vaginal dilatation is carried out under a general anaesthetic. They have a condition known as **vaginismus**. In this condition, there is an involuntary spasm of the muscles which surround the entrance to the vagina whenever any attempt is made at intercourse. Examination under anaesthesia invariably shows that there is adequate room for intercourse to take place. Surgery has nothing to offer in this very unfortunate condition because the causes are usually rather complex psychological problems which frequently relate to a traumatic experience in childhood. Infertility is bad enough, but these women are unable to even enjoy the physical aspects of love-making with their partners. Psychosexual therapy is required and it is only after prolonged, patient and sympathetic treatment by a fully trained expert that success might be obtained. If you feel that you may have vaginismus, it is essential to seek help. Your family doctor or you yourself can find out the whereabouts of your nearest psychosexual counsellor or clinic.

Cervical surgery

A very common finding during speculum examination of the cervix is a **cervical polyp**. A cervical polyp is an overgrowth of the skin lining of the canal of the cervix. It is invariably benign (not malignant) and often trouble free. Sometimes a polyp can be a nuisance because it can bleed after intercourse if it gets thumped. If the stalk of the polyp is narrow it can be simply twisted off from the cervix (**cervical polypectomy**) in the clinic (Fig. 20). It is a painless procedure. If, however, the stalk is very thick, or if there is a lot of spontaneous

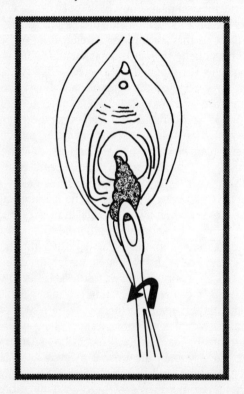

Fig. 20: A cervical polyp is grasped in polyp forceps and gently twisted until it is detached from the cervix.

bleeding between periods, or if the periods themselves are very heavy, it is then advisable to remove the polyp under a general anaesthetic. This will then also permit the surgeon to explore the cavity of the uterus to make sure that there are no other polyps within the uterus. This exploration of the uterine cavity is probably the commonest gynaecological operation performed and is known as a **D & C**, which stands for **dilatation** of the cervix and **curettage**, or 'scraping' of the uterus. The cervix is first gently stretched and the length of the uterine cavity is determined with a fine probe, known as a sound. A curette is carefully introduced through the dilated cervix and is used to explore the internal surface of the uterus (Fig. 21).

Any polyps that may be present are usually easy to remove. If there is irregularity of the inner surface of the uterus this will suggest the possibility of fibroids (Chapter seven). A D & C can reduce the

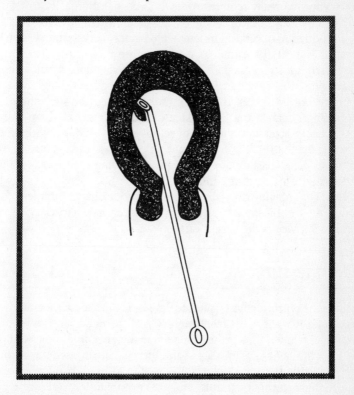

Fig. 21: An endometrial polyp is easily removed when a curette is passed through the dilated cervix.

heaviness and length of the period, remove polyps, detect fibroids or a septum, but, in itself, it is unlikely to improve your fertility.

The cervix of the uterus is covered with skin. Sometimes the lining of the canal of the cervix grows down over the cervical skin producing a bright red area called **cervical ectopy.** (This used to be wrongly called a cervical erosion because the appearance of the cervix looked raw and 'eroded'.) Cervical ectopy is extremely common and usually does not cause any problems. It can, however, produce an increased amount of vaginal discharge which you can find trying. Cervical ectopy can also become very tender and lead to pain during intercourse and bleeding afterwards. Once cervical ectopy causes problems, it is best that it is treated. If a recent cervical smear has not been taken, this should be done first. The cervix can then be cauterized. There are two types of cautery, hot and cold. Hot cautery, to be effective, really requires some form of anaesthesia. If carried out too deeply it can destroy some of the glands which are necessary for the production of cervical mucus. Cold cautery **(cryocautery)** can be carried out in the clinic without any form of anaesthetic being required. It also has the advantage of being very superficial without damaging the important mucus-producing glands. This type of cautery 'burns' the cervix in the same way as you can stick and burn your finger against the frozen side of a deep-freeze. A flat probe is placed in contact with the area of ectopy which is cooled with liquid nitrous oxide to −80°C. This freezing process is carried out for two minutes. The freezing and subsequent thawing of the cells in the cauterized area fractures the walls of the cells, thereby destroying them. The thawing does produce a watery discharge for a few days but is not troublesome. New skin grows over the cauterized zone and within six weeks the cervix can look as good as new.

Uterine surgery

When the reproductive organs are developing in a female foetus, there is a solid tube of tissue from each side of the pelvis, the lower two-thirds of which join together. This tissue then becomes hollowed out to form the cavities of the vagina and uterus. The unfused upper third on each side becomes hollowed as well to form each fallopian tube. It can be seen that incomplete fusion is going to lead to a variety of abnormalities of the uterus and vagina as well (Fig. 22).

The commonest developmental variation from the normal is the

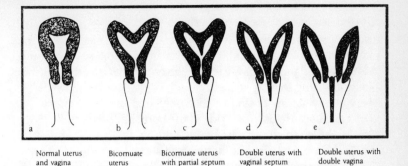

| Normal uterus and vagina | Bicornuate uterus | Bicornuate uterus with partial septum | Double uterus with vaginal septum | Double uterus with double vagina |

Fig. 22: Abnormalities of the uterus and vagina that can contribute to infertility.

bicornuate uterus (Fig. 22b) where there has been incomplete fusion of the upper part of the uterus. The uterus looks and feels heart-shaped. If not found on clinical examination, it is easily recognized with the aid of either laparoscopy or a hysterosalpingogram. When fusion is further reduced there can be a wall or **septum** which is usually incomplete and partially divides the cavity of the uterus into two chambers (Fig. 22c). Sometimes the septum is complete (Fig. 22d) so that the uterus is double and the septum can then extend partially into the vagina. When the vaginal septum is also complete this results in a double vagina as well as a double uterus (Fig. 22e). It is rare for the vaginal septum to cause any problem. The majority of women who have one don't realize it until they have been informed by the clinic. Generally, one of the vaginas only tends to be used for intercourse. Problems can occasionally arise when it comes to delivery of a baby, but the septum can usually be dealt with at the time by incising it just before delivery and then removing the remnants after the whole delivery has been completed. If the vaginal septum does cause any pain on penetration at intercourse, it is best that it is removed. This is a straightforward procedure to carry out under a general anaesthetic.

The uterine septum can, however, be associated with miscarriages. If an embryo implants onto a septum, the pregnancy is likely to miscarry as the blood supply to the placenta via the septum will be inadequate. It is pure chance as to where on the uterine wall an embryo happens to implant. Eventually it would be expected that a pregnancy with a normal implantation site would occur. I feel that the operation to remove a uterine septum (known as a **hysteroplasty**) is very rarely justified, except perhaps in the case of repeated miscarriages. The operation is a moderately difficult one to perform. It involves removing the entire mid-section of the uterus containing the septum and then joining the two halves together to form a slightly smaller but single cavity uterus.

Very rarely it can be found that only one tube and ovary has developed, because only one side of the body has contributed tissue to make these structures. The uterus with its single tube and ovary tends to be a bit smaller but that in itself should not affect fertility. If such an abnormality is found, your specialist is likely to recommend that you have an X-ray investigation of the kidneys too. The reason for this is that the development of the genital tract is closely associated with the development of the kidneys and the ureters which pass from

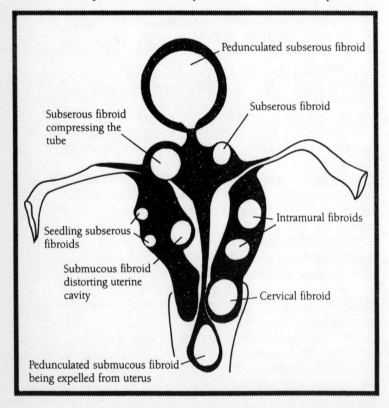

Fig. 23: The sites of possible fibroid growth within the uterus.

them to the bladder. Therefore, a developmental abnormality in one is more likely to be associated with a developmental abnormality in the other, e.g. an absent tube and ovary being associated with an absent kidney and ureter on the same side.

Fibroids are a common benign (not malignant) tumour of the muscle and fibrous tissue that make up the substance of the uterus itself. They can occur literally anywhere in the uterus from the fundus at the top, down to the cervix. They also vary in their actual position in the uterine wall (Fig. 23).

Fibroids can grow beneath the smoother outer peritoneal covering of the uterus (subserous fibroids), within the depths of the muscle wall (intramural fibroids), or beneath the endometrial lining of the uterine cavity (submucous fibroids).

The fact that you have a fibroid uterus may come as a complete surprise to you when you are told about it at the clinic. The uterus is usually found to be enlarged and sometimes considerably so. If fibroids grow rapidly, they can sometimes become massive, looking very much like a six-month pregnancy! If there is just a single fibroid, the uterus will feel smooth and enlarged. But often fibroids are multiple which makes the uterus feel very irregular and knobbly. Big fibroids can feel like a hard grapefruit with several hard apples and walnuts all stuck together!

Fibroids occur most commonly among black women and those women who have had no children by the age of 30. It's almost as if the uterus decides it better grow something if there is no baby arriving! Whether or not fibroids will cause problems, will depend chiefly upon their site in the uterus and their size.

Subserous fibroids are usually the ones that can reach a very large size but may not cause any symptoms at all. If they grow out on a stalk (when they are referred to as being pedunculated), they can occasionally become twisted causing severe pain and vomiting. A subserous fibroid that is symptom free can usually be left alone unless its size indicates that it should be removed.

Intramural fibroids do not cause problems unless they enlarge to such a degree as to obstruct by pressure the insertion of the fallopian tubes as they pass into the substance of the uterus. If they grow sufficiently large they can also distort the shape of the cavity of the uterus.

Submucous fibroids will distort the uterine cavity and so actually increase the surface area of the endometrium shed during a period. The result of this is that periods can become very heavy with episodes of flooding. This in turn can lead to anaemia and a general state of tiredness. Submucous fibroids can also become pedunculated and twist when they will cause severe pain and haemorrhage. Sometimes these fibroids can pass through the cervix and into the vagina. From a fertility point of view, submucous fibroids can interfere with the normal implantation of an embryo.

Very rarely, fibroids can occur not in the uterus but in unusual sites like the cervix. Cervical fibroids can cause pain at intercourse and if the patient is fortunate enough to get pregnant in the first place, the eventual delivery of the baby can be obstructed.

Fibroids cause infertility in three chief ways:

1. Compression of one or both fallopian tubes.
2. Distortion of the shape of the uterine cavity.
3. Interference with normal implantation.

If fibroids are small and not producing any symptoms it is best that they are left alone. They are, however, able to grow until the time of the menopause. If fibroids have been diagnosed, your specialist may wish to carry out a hysterosalpingogram X-ray to assess the shape of the uterine cavity. A new technique, **hysteroscopy**, allows the cavity of the uterus to be explored using a fine telescope, introduced via the cervix. Small submucous fibroids or polyps can be easily diagnosed and removed. In addition, it is possible to assess the internal openings of each fallopian tube into the uterine cavity. This is rather like doing a laparoscopy within the uterus.

In someone whose family is complete, troublesome fibroids can be removed along with the uterus by means of a hysterectomy. This procedure obviously would be against your best interests if you were infertile! If there is infertility or if you still hope to increase the size of your family, fibroids can be removed by an operation called **myomectomy**. In some ways this is more of a major operation than a hysterectomy, in that it is often more difficult to perform, and can involve some considerable blood loss. Because of the risk of haemorrhage during a myomectomy, specialists will warn you that sometimes the only way to literally 'turn the tap off' is to go ahead and carry out a hysterectomy. This drastic step (*very rarely* carried out) would obviously be a disaster from the point of view of your fertility, but I can assure you that it would be very much a last resort and only used as a life-saving measure.

When fibroids are very large and it is considered that there is considerable risk of haemorrhage, it is possible, after several months of treatment, to shrink the fibroids down and so reduce the possible blood loss at operation. This involves the use of a drug which is derived from the hormone LHRH (Chapter six). These so-called 'LHRH analogues' can be administered as a nasal spray five times a day when given in the form of the drug **buserilin** or as a monthly injection under the skin of the abdominal wall when given as **goserilin**. While you are on this treatment, periods will stop altogether and it will not be possible to get pregnant.

Myomectomy is a major operation and is carried out under a general anaesthetic. If the fibroids are not unduly large, the incision can be below the 'bikini line', but if they are very large, then I'm afraid you must sacrifice your perfect appearance on the beach and have an 'up and down' mid-line incision. Because of the risk of haemorrhage, it is important that cross-matched blood is available in case the need for transfusion arises.

The aim of a myomectomy is to remove all the fibroids, repair the uterus, and so restore it as near as possible to normal. Using the minimum number of incisions in the uterus, the fibroids are easily 'shelled out' of their capsules. It is important to open the cavity of the uterus in order to be able to remove any submucous fibroids that could be distorting the uterine cavity. After the fibroids have been removed, the uterus is a rather sorry-looking, floppy structure. The cavities that used to be occupied by the fibroids must all be obliterated with dissolving catgut stitches. Sometimes it is necessary to remove some of the over-stretched wall of the capsule that had originally surrounded the fibroid in order to bring about a satisfactory repair. Usually, after the myomectomy has been completed, the supporting ligaments of the uterus are very floppy and need to be tightened. This 'hitches up' the uterus and prevents it from tilting dramatically backwards.

Finally, it is important to appreciate that if after an extensive myomectomy a pregnancy should occur, there is every likelihood that a Caesarean Section will be advise as the method of delivery. This is because the incisions that have been made in the uterus may be regarded as potential weak spots which might give way when you are in labour.

Tubal surgery

Tubal problems account for at least 15 per cent of the cases of infertility, and this figure is likely to rise with an increasing incidence of pelvic inflammatory disease in the community. Public awareness of AIDS since 1986, has, for the first time, led to a downward trend in the incidence of sexually transmitted diseases. But tubal damage is not only caused by sexually transmitted infections like gonorrhoea; infection can occur after a completely normal pregnancy or can complicate a miscarriage. Infection is a well recognized complication of termination of pregnancy and can occur no matter how carefully the operation is carried out. A termination is a short-term solution to the problem of an unwanted pregnancy but it can certainly have a most unpleasant long-term kick-back. There cannot be anything much worse for a young married couple than to opt for a termination of pregnancy because a baby would be 'inconvenient' at that stage in their lives, perhaps because of their careers or mortgage commitments, and then later learn when they *desperately* want a baby that an infection related to the termination has now essentially sterilized the woman. Infection can be related to a chronic illness like pelvic TB or an acute disease like acute appendicitis with peritonitis. It can also complicate the insertion of an IUCD (intra-uterine contraceptive device), but it is difficult to be sure whether the infection is related to the insertion of the device or whether it pre-existed the insertion and was 'stirred-up' by the IUCD. For this reason, the majority of specialists and Family Planning Clinics will be reluctant to recommend an IUCD to a girl who has never had children, unless no other method of contraception is suitable. Finally, it is possible that even a viral infection in childhood may lead to this unfortunate end result.

Although infection is the chief cause of tubal obstruction and adhesion formation, adhesions commonly occur after surgery. The outer covering layer of the abdominal and pelvic organs is very delicate. Inflammation of this delicate tissue during surgery can be caused by the presence of blood, which is often impossible to avoid, the use of surgical gauze packs to hold back the large bowel to get better exposure at the site of the operation, and even just the handling of the tissues being operated upon.

It is important to remember that half of the women who are subsequently found to have blocked tubes have no significant past medical history that might indicate that there is a problem. The likelihood of a tubal problem can be suggested by a couple's history.

Case 11

Nicola had two terminations of pregnancy while she was a teenager. During the three years that her first marriage lasted, she tried to conceive but without success. After the marriage broke down, her husband remarried and his new wife became pregnant almost immediately. Nicola in turn eventually remarried, this time to a man with two children from a previous relationship. She again failed to become pregnant. The spotlight now focused itself on her. Although she had proven her own fertility in the past, she was now unable to conceive with either of her fertile husbands. Blocked tubes were found to be the cause of her infertility.

The diagnosis of tubal obstruction will in most cases be confirmed by laparoscopy. A hysterosalpingogram will at times be necessary to back up the laparoscopic findings.

If your fallopian tubes are blocked, you have to all intents and purposes become sterilized. Your chances of becoming pregnant by doing nothing are nil. With the use of skilled microsurgery techniques, fine operating instruments and non-absorbable and non-reactive suture materials, successful pregnancy rates of 30 per cent overall are possible. Obviously the degree of success will depend upon the degree of tubal damage. If there are only a few 'polythene-like' adhesions distorting the tubes, the success rate of surgery can be expected to be high. Conversely, if the degree of distortion and obstruction is severe, then the chances of surgery being successful are rather more grim. This is something that your specialist will wish to discuss with you before you make up your mind to have surgery. (This is discussed further in Chapter nine.)

One group of women with blocked tubes are those who have opted for voluntary sterilization. For a variety of reasons, a woman will sometimes request to have her sterilization operation reversed. There may have been a family disaster such as the death of her husband or of a child. She may have remarried and wish to have a baby by her new partner, or she may simply have changed her mind and bitterly regretted the original decision to be sterilized. If the request for reversal of her sterilization is because she now has a new partner, it is essential to first make sure that the new partner's semen analysis is normal. It would be ridiculous to undertake major surgery and only later find out that he was sterile! I always carry out a preliminary laparoscopy before agreeing to reverse a sterilization. This is especially important when the original sterilization method has been to remove a section of tube (Pomeroy sterilization) or performed with diathermy (a form of cautery). Sometimes one can find that either an excessively large portion of each tube has been removed or that the entire tube has been destroyed by diathermy leaving nothing to 'reverse'. It is better that this is found out by the relatively minor procedure of laparoscopy, than to carry out major surgery by opening the abdomen and then find that nothing can be done. When only a minimal amount of each tube has been destroyed, as with clip or ring sterilization, the pregnancy rate can be well above 70 per cent because healthy tube is being joined to healthy tube.

Tubal surgery is a major abdominal operation performed under a general anaesthetic. It is usual to carry out such surgery through a low 'bikini' incision.

Before deciding upon tubal surgery you will have been warned about the increased risk of ectopic pregnancy. It is always possible for an enlarging early embryo to get stuck in an area of scar tissue that has formed after surgery. Fortunately, the incidence of such ectopic pregnancies is usually quite low: less than 5 per cent of all the successful pregnancies that follow tubal surgery.

Hydrosalpinx surgery

The operation to correct a hydrosalpinx (Fig. 24a) is called a **salpingostomy**. This involves carefully opening up the blocked outer end of the tube. When the damage has been slight, the fimbrial end of the tube can open up rather like the opening of a flower. To discourage it from closing up again, the edges of the opened tube are turned slightly outwards rather like the lip of a vase. Very fine stitches are used for this. If the tube is grossly distorted, there is little point in trying to carry out a salpingostomy. In all probability, the delicate tubal lining will have been destroyed by the inflammation process, and to make the tube patent is really asking for trouble in the form of an ectopic pregnancy. It may in fact be better to remove the very badly damaged tube or simply leave it alone and hope that surgery on the opposite tube will be more rewarding. This, of course, shows the importance of having had a carefully carried out preliminary laparoscopy. Very severely damaged tubes would probably not get as far as even having an attempt at tubal surgery because the rewards would be so low.

Division of adhesions

The division of adhesions (Fig. 24b) around the tube is known as **salpingolysis** and, from around the ovary, as **oophorolysis**. The

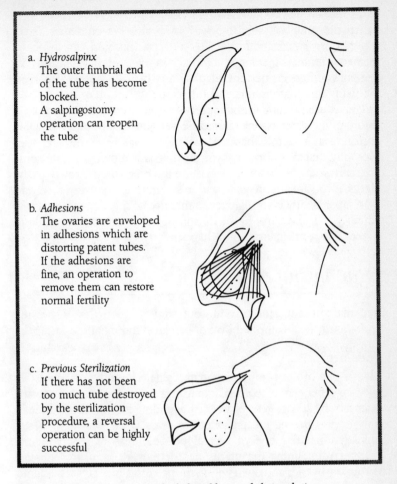

a. *Hydrosalpinx*
The outer fimbrial end of the tube has become blocked.
A salpingostomy operation can reopen the tube

b. *Adhesions*
The ovaries are enveloped in adhesions which are distorting patent tubes. If the adhesions are fine, an operation to remove them can restore normal fertility

c. *Previous Sterilization*
If there has not been too much tube destroyed by the sterilization procedure, a reversal operation can be highly successful

Fig. 24: The main categories of tubal problem and their solution.

careful removal of these adhesions can have a dramatic effect upon fertility. If the adhesion tissue is very fine, the tubes and ovaries beneath such adhesions are often completely normal and healthy. If the ovaries are enclosed in a bag of such tissue it can be seen that freeing the ovaries so that eggs have now got access to the tubes may be all that is required to restore fertility to normal. On the other hand, sometimes the adhesion tissue is very dense, almost resembling plastic. Hopefully, such cases will have been excluded by the preliminary laparoscopy.

Removal of blocked tube segment

When the tube has been blocked at its junction with the uterus, whether by sterilization (Fig. 24c) or by infection, the blocked segment of tube is first cut out and a 'join-up' (technically known as a re-anastomosis) is performed. This very delicate surgery is carried out using fine instruments and micro-surgical techniques.

After you have had a tubal operation you will be asked to keep a record of the dates of your periods so that you will be aware of going overdue. Should this happen, it is essential that you are seen promptly, first to confirm that you are pregnant and then to determine with ultrasound scans whether or not the pregnancy is safely in the uterus. If you are not pregnant within six months of surgery, a 'second look' laparoscopy is strongly recommended so that you at least know where you stand. Are the tubes still open? Is it still reasonable to expect that a pregnancy could happen?

Ovarian surgery

The main reasons for carrying out surgery upon the ovaries are endometriosis and the removal of benign tumours and cysts.

Endometriosis

This is one of the commonest gynaecological conditions, probably affecting 2 per cent of women. It may be a significant factor in causing infertility in 20 per cent of women attending an Infertility Clinic. It only occurs during the reproductive years while a woman is still menstruating. For one of several possible reasons, some of the endometrium lining the uterus has developed or been deposited within the ovaries and often within the pelvic ligaments. This 'ectopic' endometrium is active (under the influence of hormones) and is able to menstruate with the lining of the uterus. But unlike the uterus, which has a cervix through which menstrual blood can escape, endometriosis within the ovaries produces a 'period' with no way out. As a result, a blood blister forms. With successive periods the ovarian endometriosis menstruates into itself and the blister enlarges to form what is known as a 'chocolate cyst', so-called because of the dark brown colour of its liquid contents. (Doctors call all sorts of nasty things after food, but this hasn't put me off chocolates yet!)

Endometriosis typically gives you symptoms of heavy periods, period pain that often increases in severity as the period progresses, painful intercourse which can be severe enough to make you say 'Stop!', and of course, infertility. Oddly enough, the worse symptoms seem to occur when there are only tiny deposits of endometriosis present, particularly within the pelvic ligaments. Large chocolate cysts often produce no symptoms at all.

The confirmation of the diagnosis of endometriosis is usually made while undergoing laparoscopy. Black specks of endometriosis may be seen on the surfaces of the pelvic ligaments and the ovaries. There may be dense adhesions within the pelvis and ovaries distended by huge thin-walled chocolate cysts. Curiously, the tubes are virtually always open even in the most severe disease.

It is often said that the best cure for endometriosis is pregnancy, but the trick is to first get pregnant! During pregnancy the menstrual cycle is suppressed. This means that the active endometrium within the endometriosis is also forced into a state of inactivity and often regresses and disappears altogether. The treatment of endometriosis can be medical (using drugs), surgical, or a combination of both. Briefly, the aim of medical treatment is to try and create an artificial pregnancy state by stopping periods for 6-9 months. The drug used for the longest time to try and achieve this is called **danazol**. Danazol works basically by blocking FSH from the pituitary gland and so preventing a cycle from occurring. The dosage of danazol required to suppress menstruation ranges between 400-800 mg per day. The majority of women tolerate danazol very well although there can be some *temporary* side effects such as weight gain, reduction of breast size, and increased oiliness of facial skin. Very rarely, there can be moderate lowering of the voice pitch. This is said to be a permanent side effect and is an indication to stop treatment (I have only seen this on one occasion and the patient's voice returned to normal). The idea is, that after the months of FSH suppression and the drying up of all the endometriosis, upon stopping treatment the pituitary rebounds in delight, pouring out FSH, and a pregnancy follows. Some women respond well to low-dose treatment, their endometriosis disappearing within months and a pregnancy occurring after treatment stops. Others do not respond at all to high dose treatment and it may even be impossible to suppress menstruation on the maximum dose. Sometimes women are found to be completely cleared of their endometriosis and still fail to get pregnant, yet most gynaecologists will have seen a pregnancy occurring despite endometriosis. A curious condition indeed!

The newer LHRH analogues **buserilin** and **goserilin**, which can be used to shrink down fibroids and so reduce bleeding when it comes to myomectomy, can also be used to suppress menstruation in women with endometriosis. These drugs cannot be taken by mouth as they are destroyed within the stomach. Buserilin is taken as a nasal spray five times a day. Goserilin comes in a pre-loaded syringe and 3.6 mg is injected beneath the skin of the lower abdominal wall every four weeks. The continuous use of LHRH analogues switches off or 'down-regulates' the pituitary gland and so suppresses the production of FSH and LH. The big advantage is that the side effects that can occur with danazol do not occur with these drugs. Some patients will experience mild hot flushes and slight vaginal dryness.

The problem of drug treatment for endometriosis is that during the 6-9 months of treatment a pregnancy cannot occur. For this reason I feel that surgery, combined with a short course of drugs, may be best, because the time-span of treatment can be very much shorter.

If only tiny deposits of endometriosis are found with laparoscopy, I have often found it relatively easy to destroy all visible endometriosis with diathermy during the examination by making an additional tiny incision to introduce the diathermy probe. If endometriosis is more extensive, then an open abdominal operation is required. If huge chocolate cysts have been found at laparoscopy, it is useful to shrink the cysts down with 2-3 months of goserilin injections before surgery. Surgery to remove ovarian endometriotic cysts must be undertaken with the utmost care, because the big risk is that adhesions may form over the surface of the ovaries after the operation. The endometriosis must be carefully dissected out of the ovaries (which are extremely delicate structures). The opened-up ovaries must then be repaired using fine nylon sutures (stitches) to close the spaces that had previously been occupied by the chocolate cysts, and to repair the incision in the wall of each ovary. The use of such stitches — they do not create any inflammation — greatly reduces the chances of adhesion formation. If the endometriosis is severe, three months of treatment to suppress menstruation after surgery is often worthwhile.

The enigma of endometriosis remains, in that there doesn't seem to be a rule; some women will respond and get pregnant and pregnancies are also found in women who do not respond to treatment. Endometriosis causes a great deal of misery to many women, of which infertility is only a part. Endometriosis self-help groups have helped thousands of women to understand and perhaps come to terms with their condition.

Benign ovarian cysts and benign tumours

Sometimes an ovarian enlargement can be detected when you are first examined in the clinic. If it is thought that there may be an ovarian cyst present, it is usual to arrange for you to have an ultrasound scan of the pelvis to confirm the clinical findings. At other times, a cyst is only noticed when you are being examined under an anaesthetic or having a laparoscopy carried out.

Simple cysts of the ovary are quite common findings at laparoscopy and are usually insignificant. Larger cysts or solid ovarian tumours must be investigated further if only to give you the peace of mind that they are indeed benign and not malignant. It is certainly very unusual to find a malignant ovarian tumour in someone of child-bearing age.

When a large cyst or tumour is found, it is generally recommended that it is removed. This will involve an open abdominal operation. If the cyst is not too large, it is possible with careful surgery to remove it intact by literally shelling it out of the ovary. The ovary is then repaired as after removal of an endometriotic cyst. If the cyst is very large, this can produce two problems. Firstly, the fallopian tube on the side of the affected ovary may have been so badly stretched over the cyst as to be damaged and of no use. Secondly, the only way of removing really big cysts is to remove the entire ovary. Even if the cyst itself could be removed, there may not be much left of the ovary on that side.

One particular type of benign tumour of the ovary is called a dermoid cyst. This common cyst is most curious since it can contain skin, hair, teeth, and cells from almost any other organ in the body! (I have even found one such cyst which contained brain cells. I was hoping that the patient would tell me she had been having some very strange thoughts recently . . .!) It's not really surprising that the ovary can make such bizarre structures, if one considers that the egg carries the potential for making may different types of cells in the development of a baby. Dermoids can be present in both ovaries. It is, therefore, always advisable when removing one dermoid cyst (which may mean removing the whole ovary), to also split the other ovary. In 20 per cent of cases, a small dermoid is found in that ovary too; this can then be removed while preserving the rest of the ovary. If not investigated, that undiagnosed additional dermoid cyst could grow in the months ahead and might mean the loss of that ovary too one day.

There is no reason to delay trying to become pregnant after the removal of these types of benign ovarian swellings.

8

What can be done for the infertile man?

In at least 50 per cent of infertile couples there will be a significant male factor contributing to the problem. For the majority of couples, the first suggestion of this possibility will have come from the results of the initial semen analysis. These may range from a complete absence of sperm in the seminal fluid (**azoospermia**), to a major reduction in the numbers of sperm being produced (**oligospermia**). The sperm count may be normal, but the motility of the sperm may be reduced or the abnormality rate be high. There may be evidence of sperm clumping indicating the likelihood of sperm antibodies sticking the sperm together. If the white blood cell count in the samples is high, this would indicate the presence of infection.

How often I have seen the look of relief that comes over a man's face when he realizes that he has been 'cleared' as the chief 'suspect' in the 'crime' of infertility! I have found that women too are generally relieved to find out that there is no apparent male problem and would prefer themselves to be labelled as the one 'at fault'. Initially, men certainly seem to be hit much harder than their partners and less able to cope with the knowledge that they themselves are actually infertile. It's the age-old confusion between virility and sterility, the feeling that a man is lacking in something essentially male in being unable to prove his masculinity to society by getting his partner pregnant. It doesn't help if on hearing the news the woman bursts out: 'You mean it's his fault!' It's as much his fault as going bald or developing diabetes! I have frequently heard men react bitterly with phrases like: 'Well, that's it then, I'm just bloody useless; *You* can get pregnant without me; What sort of man am I if I can't even get you pregnant!' It is essential that any thoughts of blame or guilt are removed quickly. A man is not judged on his sperm count. A low or absent sperm count does not make him a failure as a human being. Indeed, there are many perversely fertile men who contribute nothing to the care of their numerous children, who expect and demand that their every need is catered for, and who make most undesirable parents. Infertility is never a question of fault.

Once a problem with the semen analysis has been found, it then becomes important to obtain a more detailed history from the male partner and also to examine him.

Medical history

In Chapter four I went into some detail on the infertility history which will have been taken from you. Of special importance relating to male infertility are specific questions about any past condition that may have affected the testicles. Obviously any history of surgery involving the testicles will be significant. Yet on several occasions I have been in the situation of having taken a full history myself and it has been only at a later appointment when the semen analyses comes back as poor that he has 'confessed' to either having had undescended testicles operated upon as a child or had a testicle removed in his teens! Significant indeed! A history of any injury or infection involving the testicles is also very relevant. Certainly infected semen will be less than fertile and it is therefore important to investigate further when a sample is reported as showing a higher than normal white blood cell count. It used to be thought that mumps was a major cause of sterility in men. It is now generally agreed that even a mumps orchitis (where the testicles are acutely inflamed and swollen) is very unlikely to cause sterility.

There are other factors that can commonly affect sperm production (**spermatogenesis**): having the testicles outside the body in the scrotum would seem at first sight to be a rather poor design feature because they are certainly more vulnerable to injury there. After all, as far as the continuation of the species is concerned, it is one of the male's most important bits! The ovaries in the female are much better protected within the abdomen (Figs. 2 & 3). However, the testicles are outside the body for a very good reason, as the temperature in the scrotum is 1-2 degrees cooler than within the abdomen. Excessive heat can dramatically reduce or even stop spermatogenesis. This means that if a baby boy is delivered whose testicles have not yet descended from the abdomen into the scrotum, he is followed-up by a paediatrician. If the testicles do not descend by the time he is 4-5 years old, it is generally recommended that they are brought down into the scrotum surgically (an operation called orchidopexy). If the operation is delayed until past puberty, he will still grow up to be a strapping young fellow because the abdominal temperature will not affect the testicles' ability to produce the male hormone testosterone. However, sperm production is unlikely to ever recover.

Some men, quite unwittingly, are regularly 'cooking' their testicles every day! The daily long soak in a hot bath, and then topping-up by adding more hot water with a lazy big toe, may seem to be the height of luxury and decadence to some. Delightful though it may be to emerge from the bath glowing like a lobster, it is not the best of ideas when it comes to sperm production. The excessive heat lulls the testicles into a long term siesta and spermatogenesis suffers as a result.

I am uncertain as to the fertility of Sumo wrestlers, whose skills I greatly admire, but gross obesity will keep the testicles in a warmer environment between the increased fat on the thighs and the overhanging folds of fat in the groin areas.

If a man's job means that he will be sitting down all day, this too will increase the warmth around the testicles. This does not mean that long-distance lorry drivers or desk workers are more likely to be infertile, but simply that it may be a factor if there is a reduced sperm count.

In Chapter four I commented upon the problems of smoking and alcohol. Smoking 20 cigarettes a day will reduce both the numbers of sperm produced and their motility. Alcohol in excess will reduce the sperm count and the production of the male hormone testosterone. It will also lead to temporary impotence.

Numerous medications can affect sperm production. Many of the drugs used in the treatment of high blood pressure and tranquillizers used for anxiety states can reduce spermatogenesis. Cytotoxic drugs used in the chemotherapy of malignant conditions and anabolic steroids can have similar effects.

Some men, by the nature of their work, are exposed to occupational risks that may reduce their fertility. I have already mentioned the problem of increased heat, but there can also be problems caused by radiation, chemicals and pesticides.

From the point of view of fertility, some couples have excessively frequent intercourse, occasionally as often as 2-3 times a day. While this may be enviable, it can have an effect on the sperm count because the demand is greater than the supply and stocks are depleted quicker than they can be replenished. It can be extremely difficult for a man with this sort of sex drive to reduce his number of ejaculations to once every 48 hours.

Over-tiredness, from long working hours can have effects very similar to those of alcohol when it comes to trying to have intercourse. It is easy to see how frustration and bitterness can result, especially if at around the time of ovulation his sole interest is to go to sleep!

Although the sperm count may be normal, there may be difficulties for him at intercourse which can account for infertility. Some men simply cannot achieve or maintain an erection for long enough to allow intercourse to take place. Others may find that ejaculation is an instant event, occurring before even penetration can occur. These very distressing conditions, **impotence** and **premature ejaculation**, can be missed completely unless you can talk to your specialist about them. He cannot guess at their existence if you assure him that all is well with regard to intercourse.

Very occasionally, some men may find that at the time of the orgasm, nothing is seen to appear. A satisfactory climax is reached but there is apparently no ejaculate. This will probably be known to the couple when they first visit the clinic. It will certainly become apparent when attempts are made to produce a semen sample for analysis. This unusual condition is known as **retrograde ejaculation**. What is happening is that sperm are being ejaculated backwards into the bladder instead of forwards along the urethra. It occurs most frequently among diabetic men or where there has been previous urethral surgery.

Examination

Some Infertility Clinics will from the outset wish to examine both partners, although I feel that if the semen analyses and the post-coital tests are normal, examining the male is unnecessary. However, it does become essential to examine every infertile man. The thought of this can make a man considerably apprehensive and actually deter him from attending the clinic. He can be reassured that the examination of the external genitalia is very rapid and painless and totally private, screened behind curtains, away from the eyes of imagined would-be fascinated on-lookers!

The areas immediately available for examination (Fig. 3) are the groin areas, the penis and foreskin, and the scrotum with its contents. The contents within the scrotum that can be easily assessed are each testicle and epididymis, and the spermatic cord containing the vas deferens which pass sperm from each testicle to the urethra and the collection of veins around each vas.

In the majority of men, nothing abnormal can be found upon

examination. Operation scars may be found in the groin indicating a hernia repair. (I can remember one patient with a zero sperm count who had a scar in each groin from a double hernia repair as a baby. I am quite sure that he also had what was effectively a vasectomy carried out on each side with each vas cobbled up with the repair!)

Sometimes the testicles are found to be very soft and small. Very rarely a testicle or a vas may be absent altogether owing to a failure of development. If a testicle cannot be felt it may mean that it is still undescended. Quite a number of men are able to draw their testicles up into the groin, or feel them pop upwards whenever they sit down. Now it may be quite useful to be able to yo-yo your testicles up and down if you are a wrestler, but it doesn't do much for fertility owing to the increased temperature around the testicles when in the groin.

Frequently examination reveals the presence of a cluster of varicose veins in the spermatic cord around the vas on either one or both sides. These collections of veins are known as a varicocele. The function of the normal veins from each testicle is not simply to carry blood away from each testicle, but also to withdraw some of the heat from the blood in the artery which they surround. When the veins become varicosed and form a **varicocele**, they also become incompetent and blood flow within them tends to slow down, thereby actually increasing the temperature. Even a small varicocele may be significant and have an effect upon sperm production.

Sometimes there can be an excess of the normal lubricating fluid around the testicle. This is known as a **hydrocele**. These collections can become quite large and therefore awkward and uncomfortable.

Occasionally there can be defects in the anatomical development of the penis itself, which can make it difficult for sperm to be correctly deposited high up within the vagina at intercourse.

The prostate gland can be a source of chronic infection. Rectal examination is the simplest way of assessing this and will certainly reveal any tenderness within the prostate and neighbouring seminal vesicles.

Further investigation

When the testicles are found to be very small, the initial investigation to be carried out will be a blood test to assess the chromosome make-up and to carry out hormone assays. Very rarely, some men can have an additional X chromosome, a condition known as Klinefelter's syndrome. Hormone disorders are rare causes of infertility, but it is a simple matter to measure FSH, LH, testosterone, prolactin and thyroid hormone levels. These may give pointers to the cause of the problem, e.g. a very high FSH and LH and a low testosterone would indicate testicular failure in a man with azoospermia. On the other hand, if there is an obstruction in the pathway that the sperm take from the testicles, such as blockage of the epididymis or vas on each side, or absence of each vas, the hormone results would be expected to be normal. The same would apply to retrograde ejaculation into the bladder.

I have already mentioned that retrograde ejaculation may be suspected if no ejaculate is produced at orgasm. Another definite pointer to this diagnosis is the fact that men with this condition are able to pass urine while they still have an erection. This is something which is usually impossible to do owing to the closing down mechanism of the bladder neck during an erection. The diagnosis is eventually confirmed by finding sperm in the urine after intercourse has taken place.

Azoospermia is usually due either to an obstruction to the outflow of sperm or to a failure of the testicles to manufacture sperm. A testicular biopsy under a general anaesthetic would show whether or not spermatogenesis was occurring normally. A normal biopsy in a man with a zero sperm count would indicate that an obstruction was the cause of the problem. Under the same anaesthetic it is possible to carry out X-rays of each vas, called a vasogram which may then indicate the site of any obstruction.

A negative post-coital test (PCT) may give a clue to the possibility of the presence of sperm antibodies, especially if the cervical mucus appeared to be of good quality. It must be remembered that an abnormal PCT may indicate an antibody problem in the male partner, female partner or both. This may be investigated further with sperm invasion and cross-over sperm invasion tests (Chapter five). If the semen analysis has shown the presence of sperm clumping, then an antibody to the sperm is likely to be responsible. When the presence of antibodies is suspected, a blood sample is taken from each partner to look for both agglutinating antibodies (the antibody responsible for clumping) and immobilizing antibodies which will reduce sperm motility. Antibodies against sperm can also be detected in the cervical mucus of women with negative PCTs and sperm invasion tests.

I have already mentioned that the presence of a high white cell count in the semen sample can indicate that there is infection present. When this occurs, a semen sample must be sent for culture. It is also important to look for a specific organism called **chlamydia** which is known to reduce the quality of sperm and is associated with infertility. It is difficult to culture and requires a special culture medium.

In Chapter five I mentioned that some clinics will assess the ability of sperm to fertilize an egg by means of the hamster egg penetration test. The idea is that if the human sperm can penetrate the specially treated hamster egg, it gives a good indication of its likely ability to fertilize the human egg.

Treatment of male infertility

Although a considerable amount of information may be learned from the possible range of investigation, at the end of the day there is often not very much of a practical nature that can be done to improve fertility and increase the chances of a pregnancy. This is especially true for the majority of cases of azoospermia. In oligospermia, however, it is obviously of some importance and general value to be as fit and as healthy as possible. The obese man should lose weight. Excessive cigarette smoking and consumption of alcohol should be reduced or even stopped. The over-worked man should attempt to adjust his lifestyle and ensure that he gets sufficient rest and relaxation. If intercourse is an extremely frequent event, it is worthwhile to slow down a bit and hopefully give sperm production a chance to catch up!

It is known that the ejaculate of semen is made up of several components, and this information can at times be of help when the sperm count is low. In the majority of men, the first part of the ejaculate is made up of sperm from the testicles and fluid from the prostate gland. The remainder of the ejaculate is fluid from the seminal vesicles and the sperm population of this component is low. This can be assessed by doing a split-ejaculate semen analysis where the first part of the ejaculate is collected in one container and the remainder in a second container. This would seem to require some pretty nifty 'footwork' on the part of the collector! In fact if the two containers, labelled I and II, are held together with a rubber band, it is a relatively simple matter to move the containers across the 'field of fire' so to speak! When the semen analysis is carried out it should show a concentrated sperm count in the first container. If this proves to be the case, this information can be applied in two ways. Firstly, it is possible to have split ejaculation intercourse. What this means is that the man deliberately bungles the 'withdrawal method' of contraception by leaving it just a bit too late, so that the first part of the ejaculate containing most of the sperm is deposited in the vagina. When there is oligospermia it is certainly worthwhile to use this method once in each cycle around the expected time of ovulation. I would not recommend it as a routine, as to withdraw at the crucial moment is not exactly fun and is really the last thing anyone would want to do at that time. The second way in which a split ejaculate can be of use, is to produce a split sample in the usual two containers, and use the first part containing the higher sperm count for artificial insemination.

With retrograde ejaculation of sperm into the bladder, it is known that there is some defect usually in the region of the bladder neck which remains open and so allows the sperm to pass in the wrong direction. One very simple manoeuvre, worth trying, is to deliberately have intercourse while the bladder is full to bursting point! In many cases the high pressure of the urine within the bladder will discourage ejaculation in that direction and hopefully the sperm will be ejaculated out along the urethra. If this should fail, treatment becomes very much more complex. An alkaline mixture is swallowed which removes the acidity from the urine. After intercourse the bladder is emptied. It is then a relatively simple matter to centrifuge the urine, retrieve the sperm and after 'washing' use them for artificial insemination.

Impotence and premature ejaculation can be helped by psycho-sexual counselling and therapy. Impotence is an extremely distressing problem to both partners. The harder the man tries and the more conscious he is of probable failure (I *mustn't* let her down this time!), the more certain it is that he will fail. Where counselling cannot help owing to a medical rather than a psychological problem, artificial insemination can be employed using the man's own sperm produced by masturbation. Premature ejaculation is probably the commonest male problem seen by psycho-sexual counsellors. It usually responds well to therapy which is aimed at increasing the man's ability to delay the moment of ejaculation.

There are a number of DIY procedures that can reduce the temperature around the testicles and so possibly improve spermatogenesis. The wearing of boxer shorts instead of tight fitting underwear will permit more air circulation around the testicles (dare I suggest a kilt?). The temperature of hot baths should be reduced drastically. There is one little gem of a treatment that I have found can produce significant benefit in about 50 per cent of the men who try it. It is called **cold water treatment**. My conversation with the man goes something like this:

'Do you have a shower that can be moved around as opposed to being fixed on the wall? (He nods slowly, his eyes narrowing with suspicion.) Well, turn it onto cold, not freezing, but cool so that you can quite happily wash your hands in it. It's important that it should be a gentle spray and not a fierce jet. I don't want the shower to rear up on itself like a cobra. Now you have to hold the testicles away from you on the other side of your finger and thumb, because they are not stupid and will be drawn back to where it's snug and warm when the cold water hits the scrotum (the horror on his face and the glee on hers is always interesting). I want you to spray the cool water over the scrotum for two minutes every morning and every evening every day! Now because sperm production takes 74 days, you have got to be doing the cold water treatment for at least this length of time if not for three months. Then you produce another sperm sample and we can see if it has done any good. The trouble with my having given you this sort of advice in front of your partner means that she will make quite sure that you do it. But it will only be fair if she gets sprayed with cold water in the process! At least you can have some fun at the same time!'

Hormone therapy

Hormone treatment for male infertility is generally unsuccessful. Apart from the rare case where there is a deficiency in the production of FSH, without testicular failure, few of the other conditions seem to respond to hormone therapy. If there is hyperprolactinaemia it is worthwhile to attempt treatment with bromocriptine. Treatment with clomiphene, tamoxifen, human menopausal gonadotrophin, human chorionic gonadotrophin, testosterone and GnRH pumps have all been tried with very limited success. A weak male hormone called mesterolone is often prescribed to men with oligospermia but again the results have been disappointing.

The same poor success rate applies to other preparations which have been used over the years. Those that have aroused the greatest interest are arginine, vitamin C, vitamin E and zinc.

Surgical treatment

When there is congenital absence either of the testicles or of each vas, there is no treatment available that can correct the situation.

If the testicles are undescended and lie within the groin, the operation of **orchidopexy** to fix them in the scrotum is worth undertaking. There is evidence that to leave the testicles within the abdomen does increase their chances of developing a particular form of malignancy. An orchidopexy performed even in childhood does not by any means guarantee that spermatogenesis will be satisfactory in adult life. A significant number of these children will later have problems with sperm production and present with infertility.

For a long time there has been debate about the benefits of operating upon a varicocele. The reason for the controversy is that there are quite a number of men with varicoceles who have normal fertility. Yet there is no doubt that some infertile men regain their fertility and get their partners pregnant after the varicocele has been treated. It is likely that the men who will benefit from treatment are those whose varicoceles can be shown by thermography to increase the heat to the scrotum. The treatments include tying off the varicocele by what is known as a high ligation and the removal of the varicocele by varicocelectomy. Both of these procedures involve a general anaesthetic, surgery, and several days in hospital. In recent years, a newer technique has been developed by employing the skills of radiologists. Using X-ray screening to view the proceedings, a fine catheter is passed via the femoral vein in the groin to the testicular vein. The testicular vein is then blocked by introducing a clotting agent via the catheter. The advantage of this technique is that it can be carried out as an out-patient under local anaesthetic. The disadvantage is that it is not universally available.

Hydroceles are worth treating surgically not only in the hope that fertility may be improved but also to remove the discomfort of an enlarged scrotum.

If a testicular biopsy shows that spermatogenesis is normal in a man with azoospermia, then the implication is that there is an obstruction to the outflow of sperm from the testicles. If a localized obstruction can be found, especially in the lower part of the epididymis or vas itself, then the microsurgery operation of **epididymo-vasostomy** can occasionally be helpful. A similar but considerably easier operation called **vaso-vasostomy**, is carried out to remove the obstruction in each vas when a vasectomy reversal is performed. The success rate of this operation with regard to a return of sperm into the ejaculate, can be as high as 80 per cent. However, the pregnancy rate, which is really what counts, may only be 50 per cent. The difference in the two rates may reflect the fact that sperm antibodies are likely to develop if the interval between vasectomy and reversal is seven years or more. It is always worthwhile to check for the presence of these antibodies before a reversal attempt is made. Another reason for the difference in the two rates is that there may of course be an as yet undetected female cause of infertility, e.g. a new marriage where the woman has never before attempted to become pregnant.

Various microsurgical techniques have been described whereby sperm are removed from the 'other side of the block' and then used for artificial insemination, but these methods are generally unsuccessful.

Treatment of infection

I have already mentioned that the presence of white blood cells in the semen sample or a tender prostate gland indicates the presence of a significant infection. Some men with infected semen have a poor quality semen analysis while others can have what appears to be a completely normal semen analysis. It is well known from in-vitro fertilization ('test-tube' pregnancy) research, that infected sperm are less able to fertilize an egg and bring about a successful pregnancy. For this reason, once an infection has been diagnosed or even assumed to be present, antibiotic treatment is essential. If a specific infection has been isolated by culturing the semen, then the appropriate antibiotic will be given. If, however, infection is simply assumed from the presence of white blood cells in the semen, then an antibiotic is chosen that could also eradicate a possible chlamydia infection.

Treatment of sperm antibodies

Once sperm clumping has occurred due to the presence of an agglutinating antibody it is very difficult to succeed in restoring fertility. In theory it is possible to 'wash' the sperm free of the antibody and then use the 'unclumped' motile sperm for artificial insemination (AIH). If the sperm numbers retrieved in this way are too low for AIH to be successful, it might then be possible to consider the couple for in-vitro fertilization.

With steroids, it is possible to dramatically reduce sperm antibody levels. This 'immunosuppression' treatment is not without its risk, and serious side effects have been reported.

Although a great deal has been written here about different tests and possible treatments, it is a sad fact that many even mildly subfertile men cannot achieve a pregnancy. The medical profession know more about female fertility than male fertility. Female fertility is a relatively easy process to stimulate as the event of ovulation is a complex but 'one off' occurence in mid-cycle. Sperm production, on the other hand, requires a continuous shop floor production line. Defects in sperm production are therefore a frequent occurrence and much more difficult to correct. It is one of the few instances when the human male is more complicated than the female!

Once a problem with spermatogenesis has been recognized, it becomes important to start discussing the various treatment options.

9

Assisted conception techniques and other options

By going to see your doctor about your infertility worries, you have already exercised your first option, namely, to do something about your problem. On the other hand, for some couples, to let Nature take its course suits them best. They are not particularly concerned whether or not a baby arrives on the scene. If it happens, it happens; if not, well, it's just one of those things.

At your very first visit to the Infertility Clinic, an initial plan of management will be presented to you with the aim of rapidly obtaining the results of basic investigations. Armed with this information, the specialist is then able to discuss with both of you the various treatment options that are relevant to your particular situation. I feel that one of my major roles in the clinic is to act as a sorting office, sifting the available information, presenting the various options, and then pointing the couple in the right direction after they have taken a fully informed decision.

When a particular treatment plan is embarked upon, the clinic should have already discussed the various options with you: it is important that you should be able to understand the reasoning behind the selection of any particular plan of action. A treatment plan must be a logical one. For example, it would be absurd for a couple in their mid-20s to think straightaway in terms of adoption because the woman was found to have polycystic ovary disease. While adoption *may* have to be considered by them one day, the correct treatment stages for them to go through will be to first try clomiphene and if that should fail, pure FSH (page 100).

In this chapter, I take several situations where there is a major infertility problem and discuss in depth the various treatment options that may be offered to you. (I am not including the vast subject of defective ovulation as this has already been fully covered in Chapter six.)

Oligospermia/azoospermia

When the sperm count is found to be persistently very low, there are obviously going to be difficulties in bringing about a pregnancy. If you have already been trying to have a baby for what seems like forever, it doesn't help or impress you very much if you are only advised to 'keep on trying, it might happen one day'. '*Might* happen' is accurate enough, but that could mean this month, this year, next year, never! What are the options?

The possible options which need to be discussed with you are:

- AIH ('Artificial Insemination by Husband') by a range of methods including IVF.
- Donor insemination.
- Adoption.

AIH

Your partner's sperm can be artificially placed either in the cervix, the uterus or directly in contact with your eggs. Now, as it happens, most men are adequately equipped with their own 'natural syringe' which deposits sperm in the upper vagina, so you might feel that there is little point in artificially doing the same thing, especially when it's not nearly so much fun! Sperm normally reach the safe haven of the cervical mucus within seconds of having intercourse. The problem is that sperm have got quite a gauntlet to run before they ever reach the egg. Out of a total sperm count in an ejaculation of say 300 million sperm, only 300 will hit the bull's-eye! Of the remainder of the sperm, a large quantity will normally trickle out of the vagina or be destroyed by vaginal acidity. Others will be 'eaten' by cells in the uterus, go down the wrong fallopian tube, or miss the egg altogether. It's a chancy business being a sperm! None of this matters too much if the sperm count is magnificent, but if the count is very low to start with, the probability is that none of the sperm will survive to reach the egg at all. If the sperm count is low or the sperm show poor progressive motility, it may seem logical to artificially deposit the sperm sample around the cervix and within the cervical canal in the hope that it might at least ensure that the sperm have a bit of a head start. Sadly, the success of this procedure is not good, and may be no better than the chances of natural intercourse. I am often asked if it would be possible to freeze multiple sperm samples to build up a respectable count and then use that for AIH. Unfortunately, freezing sperm reduces the sperm motility and as the majority of poor sperm counts have a poor motility as well, freezing samples will only make matters worse.

I am sure that you can appreciate that AIH is a very clinical and at times, quite stressful technique. If AIH is going to be carried out at all, there should at least be a reasonable prospect of success. If the sperm count is so low that it only shows an occasional sperm at high magnification (which means that the sperm count is not even a million per ml), you are really wasting your time because it simply isn't going to work.

There is a particular group of men for whom AIH is all that is required to bring about a pregnancy. For a variety of reasons, they are unable to deposit the sperm within the vagina even though their sperm counts may be completely normal. Their problems include impotence and the total inability to obtain an erection, premature ejaculation or some anatomical abnormality of the penis. These men can, however, produce a semen sample by masturbation and this can then be used for AIH.

Another small but important group of men are those who are about to receive surgery followed by radiotherapy for a malignant tumour of the testicle. This treatment is invariably started urgently, but it is usually possible for the specialist to arrange for sperm samples to be banked as an emergency (it always seems to happen on a Sunday!) with the nearest donor insemination clinic. These samples are then available for future use by the patient if required. Similarly, men who are seeking a vasectomy operation because their families are complete, may seek to 'bank' sperm as an insurance against any future disaster. This would seem to be a sensible precaution, especially for the younger man.

In its simplest form, AIH involves an appointment being made for you at the clinic around the expected time of ovulation. If ovulation has been shown to be a regular and predictable event, say with BBT charts, then it will be relatively easy to predict the time of ovulation in each cycle. You may find it easier to use an LH predictor kit (Chapter five) but it is then necessary to have the clinic facility to see you for treatment with probably only a day's notice. There is no doubt that the ideal method of detecting the correct time of the cycle is to show good egg follicle growth by means of ultrasound. You will be asked to bring with you a freshly produced sperm sample from your partner. The majority of hospitals have no facilities for a man to produce a sample in any privacy on the premises other than in the toilets which turns it into a rather sordid business. The alternative — trying to produce a sample while cramped in the confines of his parked car outside the hospital — will probably result in his getting arrested! Some enlightened clinics provide what can only be termed a 'masturbatorium', where, in a little room, behind closed doors and with the titillation of 'helpful illustrated literature', the sample can be produced in some comfort. The quality of the sperm sample is usually rapidly checked under the microscope before insemination is carried out. You will then be asked to get onto the by now familiar examination couch. A speculum examination of the cervix is made and the sperm sample is placed mainly around the cervix with a small amount instilled into the canal of the cervix. Attempts to introduce the entire sperm sample into the uterus will mean it will either all trickle out into the vagina again or, worse, will cause considerable discomfort and cramping lower abdominal pains for most of the day. You may then be asked to lie on your back for 20 minutes to hopefully ensure that sufficient sperm will reach the cervix.

In Chapter eight I referred to the technique of split ejaculation. If this shows that the sperm count in the first part of the ejaculate is dramatically higher than the remainder of the ejaculate, it then becomes very reasonable to carry out AIH using this first part.

It is possible to carry out AIH yourselves at home if the clinic provides you with the necessary equipment.

The development of in-vitro fertilization (IVF) has resulted in a method of sperm preparation that has considerable application in AIH. A sperm sample is 'washed' in culture medium. After separating the sperm from the medium, the sperm are then covered with a layer of medium and incubated. The most vigorous and motile sperm will swim up through the medium leaving the dead and less motile sperm behind. This 'swim-up' method is able to isolate the super sperm (which of course have big 'S's on their chests and red cloaks) which can be removed from the upper part of the incubated medium and used for **intra-uterine insemination (IUI)**. It is preferable that this method of AIH is carried out in a scanned cycle where the growth of the follicle is monitored by ultrasound. The same sample can be used to provide sperm for AIH just before the time of ovulation and a day later. It takes about an hour to carry out a sperm wash and 'swim-up' and it is likely that the clinic would first wish to assess a 'swim-up' test as an investigation to see if this type of treatment would be suitable for you.

The final application of AIH is, of course, in-vitro fertilization itself.

When this subject is discussed later in this chapter, it will be seen that the total number of sperm used in IVF is really very low. If a 'swim-up' test was satisfactory and AIH was unsuccessful, it may be considered that it is worthwhile trying IVF. However, there is always the possibility that on the actual day, the sperm sample will not be up to scratch or be unable to fertilize the eggs. You may very well find that the clinic will be prepared to divide the eggs, half of them to be incubated with your partner's sperm and half with donor sperm. If your partner's sperm are successful in fertilizing your eggs, then those of course will be used. But if they should fail, then you have the eggs fertilized by the donor sperm to use as a backstop rather than waste the entire IVF procedure. Obviously, the IVF clinic will spend considerable time counselling you both before embarking upon such a plan of action.

Donor insemination

We all take our own fertility for granted. We have vague, half-formed thoughts about one day producing little versions of ourselves and having a family. When a man learns that he is sterile and that there's nothing that can be done to restore his fertility to normal, the effect of this knowledge can be devastating. It can temporarily rob him of his entire perception of himself as a man. The initial acute sense of loss becomes replaced by feelings of worthlessness. He questions his value as a human being and as a husband. He feels that he has failed his wife in the worst possible way. He can even feel shame.

The suggestion of donor insemination as a possible alternative is often met with a flat rejection. Curiously enough, I find that this rejection usually comes more vigorously from his partner. She feels that she wants *his* baby, not someone else's.

Good counselling at this point is essential. Does it really matter where a baby comes from, whether it's a donor sperm or donor egg or even a donor embryo that gives rise to that baby? If I could open a drawer and take out a baby now and say to you 'Go on, take it home, it's yours,' at first you would be rather wary, but after a while when the baby began to smile and laugh and respond to you, you would be captivated. We all have an infinite capacity for loving and every baby brings its own love with it. If anything happened to the baby you would be heart-broken. If someone threatened the baby you would, if necessary, kill to defend it. Plenty of people produce babies but that in itself does not make them parents. An unwanted and unloved child has every prospect of turning into a rather undesirable member of society. But put that child into a caring environment and see the difference. A parent gives a child love, security and education, and when the time comes, points that child in the right direction and lets go. None of us own our own children. It's not our egg or our sperm that leads to our immortality. What we are and the way we behave is influenced more by the example of our parents than by anything else.

Sometimes a patient will tell me that she simply does not like the 'idea' of donor insemination and that there is something dirty about it that she finds distasteful. I put it to her that perhaps she is not being very logical. If she can accept the 'idea' of a blood transfusion which may amount ot 1,000-2,000 ml of blood which has been through several donors' brains, kidneys, back-passages and every other part of their anatomy, how much easier it must be to accept 1 ml of screened sperm that can result in a baby. At the end of the day, no one is going to force you into a decision. But the decision that you eventually reach must only be made after you have had time to thoroughly digest the fullest of information.

So in which situations may donor insemination be considered?

1. Sterile men. Their sterility may be unexplained or follow a vasectomy or radiotherapy.
2. Very low sub-fertile sperm counts that do not respond to treatment and where AIH has failed or is unsuitable.
3. Where there is a major blood group incompatibility between the couple, e.g. a rhesus negative woman may have developed antibodies to the rhesus positive blood group of her partner and any rhesus positive baby that might result from that relationship. In severe rhesus incompatibility, these babies may not survive. There is then a case for donor insemination using sperm from a compatible rhesus negative donor.
4. When a man is known to be a carrier of an inherited and very damaging abnormality and there is a substantial risk of his children developing the actual disorder itself; donor insemination may then be preferable to termination of a pregnancy should tests detect that problem in their unborn baby.
5. The mature, stable single woman who wants a child but who either does not have or wish to have a partner.

If you are seriously considering donor insemination, I strongly recommend that any discussion that you have about this should be kept strictly between you and your medical advisors. This is not because donor insemination is a stigma of some sort that you should be ashamed of, but simply to avoid some quite unexpected future distress. For example, you may find that some close members of your family will consider that donor insemination is highly distasteful or contrary to their beliefs and this could harm their relationships with your baby. I am convinced that it is best to keep the fact of donor insemination to yourselves. I am also certain that, on the whole, it is a mistake to tell the child, although I accept that this is a personal decision. A very young child can accept almost any detail about its origins, as long as there is love and security in that child's life. You may find yourselves having to answer some questions at awkward moments, such as this loud enquiry at a crowded gathering: 'Mummy, when Daddy couldn't find the seed to grow me, how *did* someone else put it inside you?' While such an incident may be embarrassing, have you considered the reaction of other children or their parents when your own child openly explains the details why daddy isn't really daddy. 'Teasing' amongst children can be mercilessly cruel. But even this is far better than for your child to learn the truth as a young adult. It's bad enough for an 18-year-old who may already be having an identity crisis to learn that he or she is adopted. At least there is the possibility of being able to trace the real mother. It's a very different matter for any adult to accept that 'my real father is an unknown and untraceable person who came out of a syringe!' If you don't want your child to know, *tell nobody*. It's not a secret that can be easily kept. If one day your teenaged donor insemination son smashes his uncle's greenhouse window with a cricket ball for the second time, imagine the reaction when that irate relative bursts out with 'You ***! You're not my nephew anyway!' He may regret saying it afterwards, but the damage has been done. If you are going to tell, tell them young. Otherwise, KEEP IT TO YOURSELVES!

Donor insemination has been carried out in the UK and many other countries for many years now and there are now many thousands of babies that have been conceived by this method. In the UK there are no laws against donor insemination, but in some countries it is still illegal. Indeed, the law is in a curious position over the status of such babies. For many years, specialists have been pressing for all babies born as a result of donor insemination to be registered as legitimate. The advice of the Warnock Committee, for example, which was set up by the UK government to investigate many aspects of infertility treatment and management, came out strongly in agreement, but its recommendations are yet to be implemented. If you have decided that nobody is going to know that donor insemination was required to conceive your baby, then stick to that. You should insist that there is no mention of this aspect of your infertility treatment on your maternity records and your joint names should be given on the birth certificate. If there are going to be major problems over the inheritance of property, legal advice should be sought. You may then find that the father will be advised to adopt his wife's baby.

There is of course, no problem if you are producing some sperm, especially if you have normal intercourse on or around the day of donor insemination. At least in theory, it may be one of your sperm that brings about fertilization, having been carried up to the egg by the millions of donor sperm.

It is useful to adopt a certain psychology in coping with the actual mechanics of donor insemination. If you are going to have to travel some distance to receive treatment, it's a bit soul destroying to go on a long tiring train journey, have yourself inseminated, turn around and go back again, arriving back home exhausted. Instead make the day into an event! 'We're off to town for the day! We're going to the zoo in the morning, then having lunch together before a spell of window-shopping; then we're rounding off with an evening meal and the theatre! Oh, and I almost forgot, there's the clinic appointment at 2.30.' You will still arrive home tired, but so much happier. That puts donor insemination into its proper perspective. It shouldn't be permitted to rule your life or to dictate your lifestyle.

So how does such a clinic run? Firstly, the majority of potential patients are referred either by their family doctors or by gynaecologists. Some clinics are only prepared to treat married couples. Other clinics will treat unmarried couples as long as there is evidence that the relationship is a long-standing one and stable. The question of whether or not single women or lesbian couples should be able to receive donor insemination has led to much debate. I personally feel that there is no reason to refuse donor insemination to the older, mature, capable, single woman, who is financially secure, and who has a sound lifestyle. It is very much more difficult for lesbian couples to receive donor insemination. One could argue that to withhold this treatment from lesbians is simply going to drive them to seek sperm from a more dubious source and also run the risk of infection.

The main area of concern to the couple who are seeking treatment is obviously going to be how the clinic selects and screens their donors, matches donors to their partners, and maintain confidentiality. Donors are often recruited from among medical school and university students. While intelligence is very important, donors must, of course, be generally healthy.

There are certain groups of men who should *not* become donors because they have an increased risk of carrying the AIDS virus. These include homosexual and bisexual men, drug abusers, haemophiliacs who have been treated with blood products in the past, men who have lived in parts of the world such as East and Central Africa, and Haiti, where the risks of catching AIDS is relatively high, and lastly anyone who has had sexual contact with any of these groups.

All potential donors must be in good health and there must not be any known inherited disorder in their families. A detailed personal history is taken, enquiry being made into the number of sexual partners they have had in the previous six months. Any past history of a sexually transmitted disease is obtained. An examination of the genital area is undertaken to exclude any obvious problem such as genital ulcers and warts, and urethral discharge. It is recommended that a urethral smear test is taken from the penis to test for a wide range of sexually transmitted organisms. After they have been counselled about the risks of transmitting AIDS, blood is taken to screen for HIV (AIDS) antibody, Hepatitis B, Cytomegalovirus and syphilis. If the HIV antibody screening is negative, a semen sample is produced and assessed for suitability for donor insemination (there will always be some men whose semen analysis will be below the high quality demanded for donor insemination). That sperm sample is then frozen and stored. Three months later the HIV screening is repeated, and if still negative, the earlier frozen sample can then be used for donor insemination. This is not absolutely foolproof as it is thought to be possible that some people who will develop AIDS will only demonstrate this fact in their blood tests many months after they have contracted the infection. The donors themselves are followed up at regular intervals, a history of any change of sexual partner being obtained at each semen donation. All samples are frozen and quarantined for three months and only used if the donors remain negative to AIDS testing.

You may worry that a donor will only be donating semen because it is a lucrative enterprise and will not admit to the clinic any change in lifestyle or in partners that may be significant. I can certainly reassure you that, at least in the UK, at the most only a small sum is offered, so there is absolutely no financial incentive to the donor to hide any facts about himself. I hope that you can also appreciate why it is so important to only receive donor insemination from a reputable clinic and not from a 'friend' or other possibly dubious source.

It also makes sense for the clinic to wish to protect themselves. It is now usual for clinics to also screen both of you for HIV antibody and Hepatitis B before accepting you for treatment. The reason for this, is, that if you were unfortunate enough to be found to be HIV positive some months after receiving donor insemination, your natural reaction would be to blame the clinic. The clinic would also naturally wonder whether you might have been HIV positive before they ever even met you. The routine testing of both donors and recipients goes some way to avoiding such a problem.

Before donor insemination, you will wish to know that the donor has similar physical characteristics to those of your partner. The ability of any particular clinic to satisfy you on these points depends totally upon the size of their pool of donors. It is generally possible to obtain a match of skin colouring, hair and eye colouring, general body build and blood group. The samples from donors of different ethnic groups are kept rigorously separate from each other. There is absolutely no chance of a mix up. One point, however, I feel I should mention: sperm do not have a religion. Religion, one could argue, is an acquired characteristic, something a particular community bestows upon an individual. However, if, for example, you should feel strongly that only a Sikh donor will be acceptable to you, and not, for example, a Hindu donor, the clinic will try and oblige — you could, however, find yourselves facing very long delays.

All information about the donor is confidential and is kept completely separate from your own records. These too are confidential documents and as such are usually stored and locked apart from normal hospital records. At the present time there is no way for a donor to learn who has received his sperm and, likewise, you cannot learn his identity. Proposals have been put forward to change the law so that children born as a result of donor insemination would have the right to trace the donor. This is being vigorously opposed by all infertility specialists, as such legislation would firstly break the essential need for confidentiality, and secondly, would greatly reduce the number of men volunteering to become donors. Clinics would certainly have no objection to keeping a register of genetic information regarding their donors, but such donors would maintain their anonymity and would still be untraceable.

Donor insemination is carried out during the fertile phase of the cycle, as close to the time of ovulation as possible. Before referring a patient for treatment, I am keen that a BBT chart is kept so that I can assess the predictability of ovulation. If the cycle is at all erratic in length, it means that ovulation will also be a very irregularly timed event. There is then a case for making sure that ovulation is predictable by using clomiphene, so that any planned insemination treatment is at least carried out on the right day. Some couples are prepared to go on a 200-mile round trip for insemination, so to go on the wrong day is not much fun. When possible, clinics will carry out 1-3 inseminations around the time of ovulation in the hope that such 'shotgun tactics' will increase the chances of success. Ultrasound scanning of follicular growth is another helpful way of accurately assessing the best time for treatment. Based on the ultrasound findings, insemination can be carried out both before and after ovulation. The stored semen sample is first completely thawed out (a process that takes seconds) from its frozen state and then, completely painlessly, is introduced into the mucus within the cervical canal. It is just like having a smear test done. It is then usual to ask you to lie on your back afterwards for 20 minutes or so. If you live a long distance away from the clinic, it is sometimes possible for the clinic to provide you with a small portable container which keeps the semen samples frozen and permits you to carry out DIY in-semination at home.

So what are the prospects of success? Freezing sperm always causes some loss of fertility compared to fresh non-frozen sperm, but the concern over transmitting AIDS means that the precautions such as screening already mentioned are essential for your protection. If there is no other factor affecting fertility, a 50 per cent pregnancy rate can be expected using this technique. Within a year of treatment, 80 per cent of pregnancies will occur, the majority being within the first six months. Donor insemination cannot guarantee that there will be a successful outcome, i.e. a pregnancy. There is the same miscarriage and ectopic pregnancy rate as for those women who achieve a pregnancy by natural means. There is also no increase in the abnormality rates among donor insemination babies.

You may surprise yourself at how you react once treatment begins. I can clearly remember one patient, who, after her first insemination, dashed back home and scrubbed herself all over! She has since had two successful donor insemination pregnancies. Another patient rang me in a state of panic because she was now suddenly facing the reality of possibly getting pregnant that month.

The baby, when it arrives, is still very much your baby. You will both be tremendously proud of yourselves and rightly so. It's also interesting just how often your partner's parents will say, 'He looks just like you when you were a little boy!'

The final option when there is a very severe male factor contributing to your infertility, is adoption. This is discussed fully at the end of this chapter.

Tubal problems

If your tubes are found to be completely blocked, you will be sterile, which sadly implies that you will not be able to have a child by natural means. You may decide that you have gone far enough, that you now know exactly where you stand and that you do not wish to have any further investigation or treatment. There is no doubt that this is the correct decision for some people, particularly if they already have children. Ideally, they may have wished to have had a larger family but would not want to go to any extreme lengths to try and achieve this goal. However, if you still wish to pursue your ambition for a family, you will need to have time to fully discuss the possible options with your specialist. The options that may be available to you include:

1. Tubal surgery.
2. In-Vitro Fertilization (IVF).
3. Adoption.

The various tubal problems and operations have already been discussed in Chapter seven. As a result of your previous laparoscopy, your specialist will have formed a good idea of the prospects of a successful outcome if you should decide upon surgery. For example, there would be little point in trying to unblock densely stuck down and damaged tubes because you would be unlikely to benefit from such surgery. You would be going through major surgery for nothing. In this situation it would make more sense to simply bypass the tubes and opt for IVF. If, on the other hand, the tubal problem only involves the removal of filmy adhesions which are separating the tubes from the ovaries, then the prospects of a happy outcome are very good. Everyone seems to want IVF and they lose sight of what surgery may have to offer. The big advantage of surgery over IVF is that if the tubes remain open and healthy after operation, you will then have an opportunity of becoming pregnant every cycle — 13 chances a year. Contrast that with IVF, where you will only have a chance of pregnancy during an IVF treatment cycle. If your resilience and indeed your purse can stand the strain, you are unlikely to have IVF more than three times in a year.

Ever since Patrick Steptoe and Robert Edwards announced to an astonished world the birth of the first 'Test Tube' baby in 1978, IVF has caught the public's imagination. Since then, several thousand babies have resulted from IVF to couples who would otherwise have remained childless. As far as the media are concerned, IVF has a glamorous image and is always newsworthy. Photographs of happy couples with twins or triplets after IVF are almost commonplace in our newspapers. The medical profession too have been partly responsible for contributing to the idea that IVF is the 'wonder treatment' that will solve all problems. Far from it, I'm afraid. Let us get IVF into perspective. *In fact, it is probably the least effective of all infertility treatments,* even though for many couples it is their only hope of a pregnancy. The overall 'take home baby rate' for each attempt at IVF is around 20 per cent regardless of what clinics may say about the pregnancy rate per egg obtained or the rate per embryo that is transferred. A rate of 20 per cent may look good when your chances of a pregnancy are otherwise zero, but don't lose sight of the other half of the equation which shows an 80 per cent failure rate! It is essential that you both appreciate exactly what you are letting yourselves in for if you are considering IVF. Without a doubt it is the most emotionally demanding of all the infertility treatments that are available.

When the prospects of success from surgery are reasonable, you may find that it is quite a difficult decision to choose between surgery and IVF. The factors that you will need to take into account will be:

- the general lack of resources to provide an IVF service near at hand coupled with the long delays in the few centtres where it is available.
- the costs of private treatment which at present are expensive.
- and perhaps most important, your age group.

If you are in your 20s or early 30s, time is still on your side, and both options are really open to you. I would then generally advise you to try surgery first and keep IVF to one side should surgery fail. On the other hand, if you are in your late 30s, time is already beginning to run out. Because the success rate of IVF falls as you approach 40 years of age, many clinics will not be prepared to offer you this treatment. It may be wisest to have your attempt at IVF while you still can and perhaps consider surgery later should IVF fail.

So just what is IVF and what is involved?

'In-Vitro' means 'in glass' and it was the media who coined the phrase 'test-tube babies'. Put at its very simplest IVF involves the removal of eggs from the ovaries, fertilizing them with sperm outside the body in the laboratory and later transferring the early embryos back into the uterus. You will see that IVF is very much more complex than this.

The first stage is to be referred to an appropriate clinic. This is usually done by the consultant infertility specialist you are attending although you may also be referred by your own doctor. Some clinics are prepared to see patients who refer themselves, particularly if they are from overseas and can bring with them the results of relevant investigations. Clinics that carry out 'assisted conception' techniques like IVF are very able to carry out all the normal routine tests themselves, as they usually also deal with the whole range of infertility problems. It is in your own interests that all the base-line investigations are carried out before you are referred, because your referral may otherwise be inappropriate. It may also save you a considerable amount of time, frustration and expense. If you decide to be seen in a non-private IVF clinic, be prepared for a very long wait indeed. From the time of referral, your first appointment to be seen may be at least two years later. If you eventually get accepted for IVF then your treatment cycle may be delayed by another 18 months to 2 years! The demand for this service, which usually receives no funding, is enormous. In an attempt to reduce the waiting time to be seen, some of these units limit themselves to only treating patients in their own health district. Others have found that the only way to generate sufficient funding to run their health service clinic, is to also operate a separate fully private service which is open to all. If, on the other hand, you decide upon private treatment, the waiting time after referral may only be a few weeks.

You will find that IVF clinics will only be prepared to treat heterosexual couples who have a stable, long-term and preferably married relationship. The clinic are not choosing to moralize over your way of life, but because the treatment can be so stressful, a reliable and stable partner is essential. Furthermore, the successful results can mean a multiple pregnancy and for this you will definitely need each other's support.

When you are seen together for your first consultation at the IVF clinic, a full history is taken and an examination is carried out. The results of all your previous tests are studied. Frequently there can be omissions such as screening for Rubella. (I can think of nothing worse

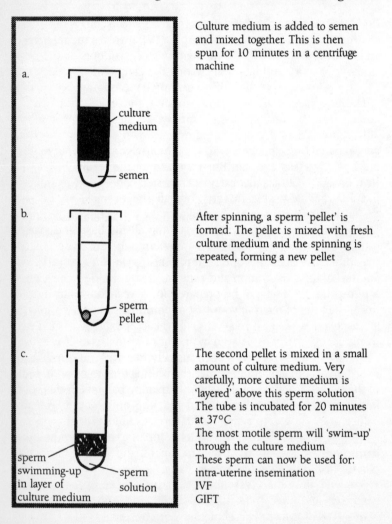

Culture medium is added to semen and mixed together. This is then spun for 10 minutes in a centrifuge machine

a.

culture medium

semen

b.

After spinning, a sperm 'pellet' is formed. The pellet is mixed with fresh culture medium and the spinning is repeated, forming a new pellet

sperm pellet

c.

The second pellet is mixed in a small amount of culture medium. Very carefully, more culture medium is 'layered' above this sperm solution
The tube is incubated for 20 minutes at 37°C
The most motile sperm will 'swim-up' through the culture medium
These sperm can now be used for:
intra-uterine insemination
IVF
GIFT

sperm swimming-up in layer of culture medium

sperm solution

Fig. 25: The 'swim-up' test, the method of assessing sperm viability before IVF treatment.

than to succeed with IVF and then contract Rubella in the early weeks of that pregnancy.) Patients may even be referred who have never had a laparoscopy or a semen analysis carried out! This illustrates the advantage of referral by an infertility specialist. There are a number of additional investigations that the clinic will need to have the results of before embarking upon a cycle of treatment. These include HIV, Hepatitis B screening, and sperm antibody tests on both of you, as well as a detailed assessment of the sperm themselves. This takes the form of the 'swim-up' test mentioned earlier. This important test (Fig. 25) gives information regarding the suitability of your partner's sperm and the likelihood of fertilization being successful.

Depending on which technique the clinic use to retrieve the eggs from the ovaries, a preliminary ultrasound scan may be carried out to determine the accessibility of your ovaries.

The clinic will explain in detail to you exactly what is involved in IVF and what the aims of the procedure are. Obviously any questions that you have will be answered. Most clinics will also provide you with written information or a booklet which clearly explains the treatment programme of that clinic. More and more centres are now also providing the services of a counsellor, so there is usually someone that you can contact even out of hours, if you should suddenly have a query regarding your treatment.

The aim of the initial fertility drug stimulation in your IVF treatment cycle is to stimulate many eggs to become mature together instead of the single egg that would result in a natural cycle. In this way more eggs will be available for fertilization and so increase the chances of success. Clinics will vary in the way stimulation is carried out. Many clinics will nowadays first completely suppress the action of your own pituitary hormones by 'down-regulating' the pituitary gland with the LHRH analogue buserilin. The buserilin is continued until the eggs reach full maturity. Once a period starts you then get in touch with the clinic who will give you the all-clear to start your egg stimulation treatment the next day. The drugs used are usually a combination of clomiphene for five days and injections of either human menopausal gonadotrophin (HMG) or pure FSH. The progress of the growth of the egg follicles is monitored closely by ultrasound and by hormone assays which measure the rising oestrogen level in blood or urine samples.

When the leading follicle reaches maturity (17 mm in diameter), which is usually around day 10 of the cycle, you are given human chorionic gonadotrophin (HCG). This injection is important for the final stages of maturing the follicles. The HCG injection must be timed for between 33 and 36 hours before the planned time of egg retrieval. Since most egg retrievals are done in the morning it means that the HCG will need to be given late at night or even in the early hours of the morning. Now doctors do not particularly welcome this aspect of the treatment but your local hospital may be helpful. However, DO NOT LEAVE THE ARRANGEMENTS FOR THIS TO THE LAST MINUTE! To avoid panic in the event that your local hospital may initially refuse to help, get this sorted out well in advance. The IVF clinic can usually help you if required.

When the great day dawns, make sure that you can get to the clinic in time. If long distances are involved, give some thought to the idea of travelling up the day before and spending the night near to the clinic. Most clinics will be able to recommend suitable accommodation in their vicinity. You will want to avoid the distress that occurred to one of my patients, who, while travelling down to London on the morning of her egg retrieval day, got caught up in a ten-mile traffic jam. She had already ovulated by the time she eventually arrived at the clinic.

On your arrival at the clinic the process of egg retrieval starts. There are essentially two ways in which this can be carried out, and very occasionally both methods will be used. The most commonly used method nowadays is by ultrasound guidance or UDOR (Ultrasound Directed Oocyte [egg] Recovery). This simple procedure is carried out under local anaesthetic or mild sedation. It is rare that a general anaesthetic is required. It also has the advantage that you and your partner can stay together the whole time. A fine needle is guided by ultrasound into the mature follicles which can be clearly seen on the ultrasound screen. The ovaries can be reached by several routes, either through the abdominal wall and full bladder, via the urethra and full bladder or, perhaps most easily, via the vagina (Fig. 26), which is by far the most comfortable as the bladder can then remain empty. The egg is gently sucked out of the follicle along with the follicle fluid contents. Quite regularly the follicle will need to be 'flushed' several times with a special culture medium solution before the egg is finally recovered. In this way every follicle that can be seen in each ovary is aspirated. Clinics frequently have the ultrasound screen positioned in such a way that both of you can see what is happening. Believe me, it is exciting every time the embryologist, who examines the fluid drawn from each follicle, announces 'I've got another egg.'

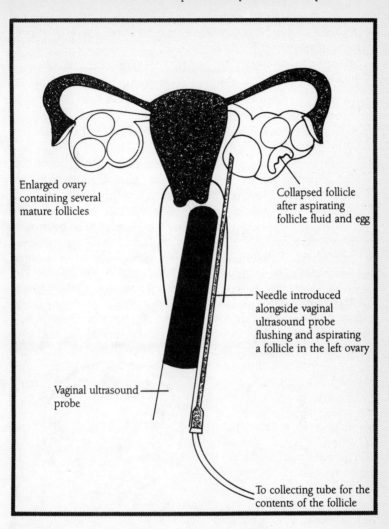

Enlarged ovary
containing several
mature follicles

Collapsed follicle
after aspirating
follicle fluid and egg

Needle introduced
alongside vaginal
ultrasound probe
flushing and aspirating
a follicle in the left ovary

Vaginal ultrasound
probe

To collecting tube for the
contents of the follicle

*Fig. 26: Eggs can be retrieved using Ultrasound Directed Oocyte Recovery
(UDOR) by the vaginal route.*

The second method of retrieving eggs from the ovaries is by
laparoscopy but this usually requires a general anaesthetic. This is
one reason why it is not used so frequently. It also requires that the
ovaries can be clearly seen to get access to them. Often when there
is tubal disease the ovaries are stuck down in the pelvis and can really

only be reached by ultrasound using the vaginal route.

As each egg is recognized, the embryologist places it in culture medium, which is a specially prepared solution that maintains the growth of the egg. It is incubated in this medium for 2-24 hours depending upon its maturity. The eggs require incubation because they were taken from their follicles prematurely, before the time that they would have naturally ovulated. This time needs to be made up so that they can reach full maturity before they are exposed to sperm and, hopefully, are fertilized.

When the eggs have been obtained, your partner will be asked to provide a semen sample for preparation. You will have abstained from intercourse for several days so as to ensure that his sperm count is sufficiently high. As an insurance policy, the clinic may have already frozen an earlier semen sample, just in case for one reason or another he cannot perform on the day. The freezing process will, however, have reduced the fertility of that particular sample. The sperm are then prepared for action as described earlier in the 'swim-up' test. The sperm are then incubated in culture medium similar to that used to incubate the eggs. This incubation of the sperm increases their ability to fertilize the eggs.

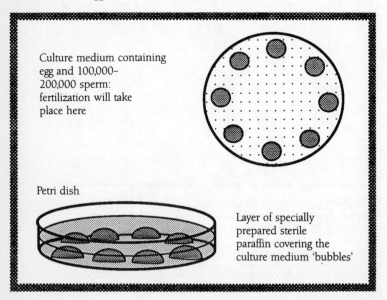

Culture medium containing egg and 100,000–200,000 sperm: fertilization will take place here

Petri dish

Layer of specially prepared sterile paraffin covering the culture medium 'bubbles'

Fig. 27: Making the 'test-tube' baby: eggs and sperm are incubated in culture medium for 12–15 hours.

When the eggs are considered to have reached maturity, they are isolated in a bubble of culture medium and 100,000-200,000 sperm are added to each egg. Up to eight of these bubbles of culture medium containing eggs and sperm occupy a small flat plastic dish, called a petri dish, so it's not actually a 'test-tube' (Fig. 27). All the eggs obtained will be incubated with sperm in this way for between 12-15 hours, the time taken to achieve fertilization, depending upon the maturity of the eggs.

After the eggs have been retrieved and you have fully recovered from any effects of mild sedation, you may return home. You will be asked to contact the clinic on the second day after egg retrieval when you will be told firstly whether or not fertilization has occurred and secondly, whether at least one embryo is beginning to develop satisfactorily. During this period, IT IS ESSENTIAL THAT THE CLINIC CAN CONTACT YOU BY TELEPHONE AT ALL TIMES.

Two to three days after egg and sperm incubation, you will be asked to return to the clinic to have up to three or four of the best embryos transferred back into the uterus. Before this is done, you will both be invited to view the embryos under the microscope — really quite something after everything you have been through together (Fig. 28).

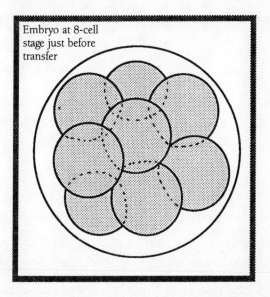

Embryo at 8-cell stage just before transfer

Fig. 28: After culturing, if all is well, the eggs should fertilize and begin to develop.

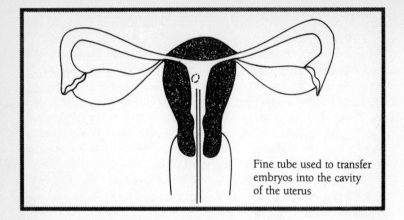

Fine tube used to transfer embryos into the cavity of the uterus

Fig. 29: Embryos are transferred, via a catheter, to the inside of the uterus, hopefully to implant there.

The transfer itself is a painless procedure taking only a few minutes. Again, you may require mild sedation. A fine tube is inserted into the cervix and the embryos are gently injected into the cavity of the uterus (Fig. 29). You will have already discussed with the clinic the number of embryos to be replaced. It is usually recommended that no more than three embryos are replaced unless in exceptional circumstances, such as several previously failed attempts at IVF. The pregnancy rate does not appear to increase significantly if more than four embryos are transferred. The risk, of course, of replacing many embryos is that a multiple pregnancy can result. The fate of the unused embryos that were not replaced will also have been discussed with both of you before your actual treatment cycle. If the clinic has the facility to freeze spare embryos to save for a future attempt then this should be done. Only embryos that appear to be dividing normally are chosen for this.

After the embryo transfer, you can return home after a short rest. It is generally recommended that you should then lead a normal but not too vigorous lifestyle and that intercourse should not take place during the remainder of the cycle.

One week after the day of egg retrieval, a blood sample will be required to measure your progesterone level. Some clinics will on this day give additional hormone support, either in the form of a further HCG injection or progesterone vaginal pessaries for a week. There is some evidence that HCG may actually rescue a failing corpus luteum, and permit a pregnancy to continue.

This is the hardest time of all. The waiting. If you have not had a period 16 days after retrieval, a blood test will hopefully be able to detect the pregnancy hormone beta-HCG.

Perhaps now you can appreciate the stresses of IVF. There are so many hurdles to overcome in the treatment cycle. Will the follicles grow? Are the sperm going to be alright? Will there be mature eggs to retrieve? Will the eggs get fertilized? Will at least one embryo appear to be developing normally? Will the transfer be alright? And oh, please, please, please, will it work? You can understand why some women, even when their treatment has been successful, will say 'Fantastic, but I wouldn't do it again!'

So just what is the success rate of IVF? An average of 6–8 eggs can be obtained at each egg retrieval attempt. Not every follicle aspirated will have an egg that can be found, in spite of repeated 'flushing' of the follicle, but an egg should be found in 80 per cent of the follicles. It is very rare to find not a single egg. Once incubated with sperm, not every egg will fertilize but fertilization rates of around 95 per cent can be expected. If only one embryo can be transferred, the pregnancy rate is 10 per cent, for two embryos 20 per cent and for three embryos 30 per cent. The big discrepancy between the high rate of fertilization and the low pregnancy rate is due to problems with implantation of the embryo. The embryos do not arrive in the uterus at the natural time of the cycle and certainly not by the natural route. Methods are constantly being sought to provide the ideal environment for the embryos so as to improve the chances of successful implantation.

Once an IVF pregnancy is established, there is still the risk of miscarriage and this risk is certainly increased when there is a multiple pregnancy. There is, however, no evidence to show that your IVF baby has any greater chance of abnormality than if you had conceived naturally.

When IVF fails, as it will do, sadly, for the majority, 'disappointment' is a mild way of describing your reaction. You will have been through so much and have got nothing from it. But at least it will have been a marvellous achievement to have got the eggs fertilized. This fact should buoy you up for another attempt in the future. If spare embryos have been frozen, there is about a one-in-three chance that they can be thawed out successfully and replaced in the future.

If both surgery and IVF should have failed you, there may still be the option of adoption which is discussed at the end of this chapter.

Unexplained infertility

To be told that you have 'unexplained infertility' (Chapter five), is a very frustrating situation for you to be in. You may even feel that it would be easier to cope with if there was something definite that was wrong. But when no cause at all can be found to explain your infertility, there is at least always the prospect that a pregnancy might one day happen. There is certainly no chance of that if your tubes are hopelessly blocked. You will in that case have found your 'something wrong', but apart from surgery, only IVF can give you the possibility of success and there is a limit as to how many attempts you will be able to cope with or afford.

So what are the options?

1. Do nothing and hope.
2. Intra-uterine insemination.
3. Assisted conception techniques: GIFT
                                    IVF
                                    ZIFT
4. Adoption

Intra-uterine insemination (IUI)

IUI is creating a lot of interest. The aim of this treatment is to ensure that in every cycle the chances of your conceiving are as high as possible. The cycle is stimulated either with clomiphene or human menopausal gonadotrophin (HMG). The growth of the follicle is monitored on ultrasound. When the follicle has reached 16 mm in diameter, your partner produces a semen sample which is prepared by the usual 'swim-up' method (Fig. 25). The most active sperm that have swum-up through the layer of medium are carefully removed. The quality of these sperm is checked by microscopy. On that day, a third of the sample is very gently and easily injected into the uterus using a fine quill. You may be asked to rest in the clinic for 20 minutes or so. The next day, this is repeated and you are given HCG to bring about ovulation. On the following day, the ultrasound scan is repeated to make sure that you have now ovulated. This is easy to detect as the large follicle seen two days earlier will have collapsed. IUI is also carried out on this day. A week after the HCG injection, blood is taken to measure your progesterone level. So what has been done, is that in a very controlled cycle, the most motile sperm that your partner can produce are placed within the uterus. Although this will involve you in several visits to the clinic, you can see that it is certainly not as intensive as IVF. Pregnancy rates in the region of 30 per cent are being reported, the same as for normal fertility.

GIFT

With the establishment of IVF, and the skills that are involved in egg retrieval and sperm preparation, a number of related methods of assisted conception have been developed. The most important of these is GIFT (Gamete [sperm or egg] Intra-Fallopian (into the tube) Transfer). In the GIFT technique, sperm and eggs are transferred together into the fallopian tubes, thereby allowing fertilization to occur naturally. The resulting embryo can then arrive in the uterus at the correct phase of the cycle allowing implantation to occur. The essential requirement, of course, is that at least one of your fallopian tubes is 100 per cent healthy and patent. GIFT is, therefore, rather like a successful match-making service, ensuring that the participants at least get to the stage of being introduced to each other. What they do then is up to them!

The preliminaries are identical to those for IVF and include fertility drug treatment to bring about the development and maturity of several egg follicles, and the same techniques of sperm preparation. The timing of the HCG injection is the same as for IVF. The retrieval of the eggs is by the laparoscopic method so this will involve your being admitted to hospital, either the day before or on the morning of retrieval. You will be asked to abstain from food prior to your general anaesthetic, and, that morning, your partner provides a sperm sample which is prepared once again by the 'swim-up' technique. At laparoscopy it is a simple matter to view your ovaries, usually considerably enlarged by all the mature follicles within them. Two additional puncture sites are made, one on each side of the lower abdomen, to allow for the insertion of a special follicle-aspirating needle. While observing through the laparoscope, this needle is passed directly into the follicle, the contents of which are gently sucked out. The follicle is then 'flushed' with specially treated culture medium which is in turn sucked out into a collecting tube. Sometimes as many as four flushes are required before an egg is eventually located by the assistant who is checking the contents of each 'flush' under the microscope. In this way, every follicle seen is emptied of its contents. In most treatment cycles, there are usually many more eggs than required. The four best and most mature eggs are chosen for transfer.

A small quantity of the 'swim-up' fluid containing 100,000–200,000 sperm is drawn up into a very fine catheter tube followed by two of the eggs. It is usual to leave a little air bubble between the sperm and eggs in the catheter. Through one of the two lower abdominal incisions, a delicate forceps-like instrument is inserted which is used to grasp the fallopian tube in such a way as to cause no damage to the fimbrial end. These grasping forceps are now required to keep the tube steady, so that a fine 'guiding' cannula tube which has been introduced through the second abdominal puncture site can be passed directly into the open fimbrial end. The catheter containing the sperm and two eggs is passed down this cannula until a 2 cm

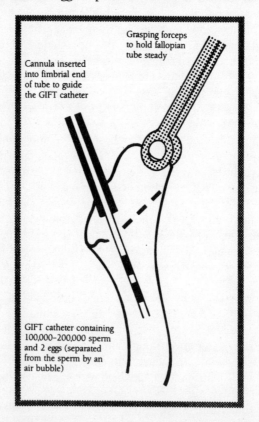

Fig. 30: The principles of GIFT (gamete intra fallopian transfer): eggs and sperm are introduced, via a special catheter, into the open end of the fallopian tube.

length has entered the tube (Fig. 30). The sperm and eggs are then injected. The catheter is removed and checked under the microscope to confirm that the eggs are no longer within it. This procedure is then repeated on the other side.

Later that day, or by the next day at the latest, you should be allowed home. The follow-up is then identical to the management of IVF.

There is no doubt that GIFT is most successful in couples whose infertility is truly unexplained. The 'take home baby' rate should be in the order of 30 per cent. If, as often becomes apparent when carrying out the initial 'swim-up' test, there is a hitherto unidentified male factor, then the success rate of GIFT is virtually halved.

GIFT versus IVF

There is no doubt that to set up an IVF service is an expensive business and certainly beyond the resources of most general service hospitals, certainly in the UK. Even the majority of UK teaching centres, for example, are unable to adequately fund IVF under the national health service. It is a different matter with GIFT. A lot of the necessary equipment is there already and the remainder is relatively inexpensive. It is not essential to have a large and expensive-to-run team of individuals to carry out the procedure. Laparoscopy is a skill taught to all gynaecologists during their training years. Any specialist who is familiar with the instrument can rapidly learn the techniques of follicle aspiration. Ultrasound skills are usually available for the maternity services and it is not difficult to extend this to the monitoring of follicle growth during a treatment cycle. The upshot of all this, is that GIFT is more likely to be readily available than IVF. GIFT is therefore likely to be used for unexplained infertility, male factor problems, and other problems such as endometriosis. The alternative choice of IVF is probably not going to become widely available, except in the private sector.

If you are being referred to an assisted conception clinic capable of carrying out both GIFT and IVF, you may be surprised to find that some centres will recommend that your unexplained infertility is treated with IVF as the first line of management. At first sight this will seem curious, as you haven't got a tubal problem and the success rates of GIFT would seem to be higher than for IVF. So why will some centres offer IVF before GIFT and vice versa? Are there advantages of one technique over the other?

The big advantage of GIFT over IVF is that once eggs are fertilized, the chances of successful implantation are high. This is because the embryos pass down the length of the tubes and enter the cavity of the uterus in the same way as a naturally conceived pregnancy. But there are some definite disadvantages too. When the eggs and sperm have been placed into the tubes, everything that then follows is hidden. If a pregnancy does not result, is it because fertilization did not occur, or was there a problem with implantation? What does one do with the spare eggs that are not used? In centres that can only offer GIFT, they are thrown away, which is not in your best interests. If the facility were to be available, these spare eggs could be fertilized and the resulting embryos frozen and stored for you, in case they are required by you in the future. Spare eggs could also be used for egg donation in the same way as sperm can be used for donor insemination.

If you have had treatment with GIFT and it fails, should you repeat the attempt? Should IVF be tried instead? Is a GIFT failure perhaps due to a problem with the ability of your partner's sperm to fertilize your eggs? It is for this reason that some centres will opt for IVF as their first choice of treatment in unexplained infertility. The clinic will then have proof that fertilization is possible. Another advantage of IVF is that only the best embryos will be used for transfer, and it is not uncommon to see an abnormal embryo; one for example, that has been fertilized by more than one sperm. Such an embryo would not be suitable for IVF and would be thrown away. Spare embryos can also be frozen for future use.

Lastly, from both a practical and financial point of view, the IVF clinic can usually function without requiring you to be actually admitted to hospital.

ZIFT

To my mind, ZIFT is the ultimate ideal treatment for at least 50 per cent of infertile couples should all else fail. ZIFT stands for Zygote (an early embryo) Intra-Fallopian Transfer. Instead of eggs and sperm being transferred into the tubes, three very early embryos are transferred instead. This seemingly complex treatment combines the best features of IVF and GIFT. It has the advantage that IVF offers, of confirming that the eggs have been fertilized, and the advantage of the higher implantation rate of GIFT as the embryos will arrive naturally within the uterus and have a chance of implanting naturally. The essential requirement, of course, is that your tubes are patent.

What's involved? Initially an IVF programme is followed. On the appropriate day, eggs are retrieved by ultrasound and after maturation are exposed to sperm. By the next day, there should be evidence of fertilization. The IVF process now stops and switches to GIFT. A laparoscopy is performed and the three most promising embryos are transferred into the fallopian tubes.

It is surprising that more assisted conception units do not carry out ZIFT. It is not much more complicated than either IVF and GIFT alone, and a higher success rate could be expected.

The final option for unexplained infertility is the possibility of adoption which is discussed at the end of this chapter.

Premature menopause and ovarian failure

Very occasionally it can happen that your ovaries run out of eggs at a much younger age than is usual. When this occurs, your periods will stop and you will enter a premature menopause. Hormone profiles will show very high FSH levels and rock bottom oestrogen levels because the pituitary gland is pouring out FSH in an attempt to stimulate the ovaries to work properly, which, sadly, they are no longer able to do. Another situation that will result in ovarian failure is when the ovaries have had to be surgically removed. This may have been required for a combination of problems such as one ovary being removed for severe endometriosis, and later the other ovary requiring removal, say, for a twisted ovarian cyst.

Until the development of IVF, there was nothing that could be offered to you in this situation. Adoption would have been the only available option. When it was found that there would often be spare eggs available from IVF and later GIFT treatments, the concept of egg donation was developed. This is a treatment option which the majority of the ethical committees attached to IVF units are happy for their units to undertake. It is, after all, no different from semen donation. It is interesting how frequently women undergoing such treatment are prepared to donate left-over eggs. Perhaps it is because they have known personally the anguish of infertility and wish to do everything possible to help other couples. However, as for donor insemination, it is best that the eggs come from an unknown donor. Often women in this situation have had the offer from a sister or a very close friend to donate eggs. This is always potentially fraught with difficulty as there is the risk of later interference from the donor in the child's upbringing. If donor eggs are to be used, your uterus will need 'priming' with hormone treatment before it is ready to accept the embryos. The donor eggs are fertilized with your partner's sperm.

Embryo transfer is carried out as for IVF.

Adoption

If it becomes clear that you are not going to be able to have children
of your own, the possibility of adoption is always an option to be
carefully considered and fully discussed. The majority of couples
who wish to adopt are at least initially thinking in terms of a baby,
but this wish is rarely fulfilled. The demand for a baby is generally
about 100 times greater than the supply. The reduction in numbers
of these babies is due to several factors. These include better
contraception with wider use of the Pill, easier access to termination
of an unwanted pregnancy and the fact that if a single girl should
decide to continue with a pregnancy and then keep her baby, it is
nowadays socially acceptable for her to do so. This has therefore
changed the adoption scene considerably. Couples who realize that
the adoption of a baby is going to be unlikely, are nowadays readier
to apply for the adoption of an older child or sibling group such as
a brother and sister, or a handicapped child who has 'special needs'.
It is very important that you consider adoption from the correct
standpoint. Adoption services are not in existence to provide the
infertile with children that they cannot have themselves. *The aim of
adoption is to provide a family for a child who cannot be brought up by
its own parents.* THE NEEDS OF THE CHILD ARE THEREFORE PARAMOUNT.

Because there are so many would-be adopters of babies, the
adoption agencies find that they have a large pool of people to choose
from. Apart from the legal requirement of being over the required
minimum age of 21, the adoptees of a baby must in general be married
couples who have a stable relationship, having been married for at
least three years. Understandably, the agencies will wish to place
babies in younger families. By the time you have been through the mill
of various infertility treatments and options, you may very well find
that you have aged yourselves out of an acceptable age-group. Once
either of you reach the age of 34, adoption of a baby will become
improbable. Agencies will however vary in their individual rules on
the age question. You will find that when it comes to considering your
application for the adoption of an older child or any child in the
'special needs' group, the requirements made by the agency are less
rigid than for the adoption of a baby. It is even possible for the stable,
mature single person to adopt a child from this group. Remember that

the main objective of the adoption agency, is to find the best family placement that will suit the needs of a particular child.

Once you apply for adoption, the agency will expect you to be completely committed to this and not try to 'beat them to it' with yet another go at IVF. I used to think that this was very unfair and that the agencies had no right to impose such a restriction upon couples. Surely, I thought, it is nobody's business but their own what they do, as long as they stop all treatment by the time they are fully accepted for adoption. I assumed that the agency would be pleased for a couple who managed to get pregnant themselves while waiting to adopt because this would release a baby to another couple. I was wrong. They would not be pleased at all. And I have partly changed my mind. Firstly, I have had the opportunity of direct contact with my own local adoption agency and now appreciate the amount of time, effort, discussion, and paper-work that goes into the visiting, interviewing and approval of prospective couples seeking to adopt. The agencies have sufficient couples who wholeheartedly wish to adopt and simply cannot afford to lose the time to couples who are regarding adoption as a last resort and only a third rate option. Secondly, I have had the disconcerting experience of being informed by a patient just as she was going off to a donor insemination clinic for her routine mid-cycle treatment, that 'I'm getting my adopted baby next week!' That certainly brought home to me the need for a commitment long before the event occurs.

The one fact that I find hard to accept is that agencies are completely within their rights to go through all the necessary screening stages, keeping a couple's hopes alive, and then at the end of the day be able to refuse to accept them for adoption *without giving any explanation*. If this happens to you, the effect is shattering. You will feel like a criminal who has been judged without a jury. You will think that there must be something very wrong with you or your marriage that has made you in some way unsuitable to be considered for parenthood. Not only have you failed to become a parent because of your infertility, but you will also feel that you have failed in the eyes of the agency to be even suitable as a parent. What may irritate you further is the fact that the majority of the social workers who assessed you were probably young and single, without experiences of their own in the establishing of a family. You will feel 'Who the hell were they to judge us!' Your hurt and indignation are understandable as there is no vetting of the fertile if *they* choose to have children. To make matters worse, your being turned down may have been due to an understandable reluctance on your part to stop all fertility treatment, or to not being happy about giving up your career when you actually adopt. If you have had some chronic illness in the past, or if there have been any emotional disorders in either of you, that can be enough to make you undesirable in the eyes of the agency. BUT YOU WILL NEVER KNOW!

I do feel that an explanation of some sort is due to you, in the same way that a specialist will explain his reasons for refusing to reverse your sterilization or to carry out IVF. You may not agree with the reasons given and feel that you have been cheated out of something to which you are entitled, but at least you have received an explanation. I am sure that there is some way in which a couple who have been turned down for adoption *after* being screened, can be given an adult explanation for the refusal. It may be hurtful and seem to be very unfair, but it would be better than wondering what awful thing has been found which has denied you the chance of adopting.

When it comes to finding suitable homes and families for babies of other ethnic groups than your own, I find it sad that their own communities do not seem to want them. It is easy to follow the reasoning of these communities but I feel that it is often based upon wrong assumptions. Since 1975, I have had a lot of contact with the Asian community in Leicester where I work, one of the largest in Europe. Yet I have found only two Asian couples in that time who have been interested in and succeeded in adopting an Asian baby. The reasons behind the community's reluctance to adopt are twofold. Firstly, because it is a very close knit and family conscious society, the young couple are very worried about the acceptance of an 'outside baby' by their immediate family and friends. If you are in this situation, you would be concerned that such a child might be rejected. I am sure that this fear is groundless. There may be some members of the older generation who will disapprove, but in 20 years time they will be dead and if you listen to them and follow their advice you will have been denied the experience of parenthood. A baby is a baby. Who is going to be able to resist any little one once they start smiling and reacting and returning love? The second worry is, that if, say, you adopt a baby Asian girl, she may one day have difficulty in marrying the person of her choice. Her potential future in-laws may wish to know details of her background, and apart from the potted history that has been given to you by the adoption agency, you will not be able to give one. But the Asian community is already changing. I am sure that any adopted daughter will be judged on her upbringing, education, and her social skills and behaviour, rather than who her genetic grandfather was. As a final reassurance, because these communities are relatively small, the adoption agencies will undertake not to place a baby for adoption in the community that it originated from. The various agencies do have links with one another and are able to place these babies in different parts of a particular country.

Perhaps even worse, is the fact that for theoretical reasons and reasons of policy, the white community cannot easily adopt non-white babies and children even if they wish to do so. The evidence against inter-racial adoption is poor and seems to theorize about the importance of identity and culture. But this is to lose sight of the main aim, which must be to find these children families and not condemn them to institutions. I was delighted when Joan Lestor, the English MP, set up the 'Children First' campaign whose aim is to get every child out of care and into a family regardless of its colour or race.

Adoption from overseas

Owing to the difficulty in adopting a baby, many couples have turned to the possibility of adopting a child from another country and have been successful. Inter-country adoption can be almost as frustrating as your original infertility management. There is no agency which exists to help you, although there are useful contacts to be made through the various associations for the childless (page 210). Through their contacts you may be put in touch with people who have succeeded and who understand the procedures and can advise you upon the correct approach. You will need to take all the responsibility yourselves for the necessary letter writing and comparatively large amounts of documentation that are required. There are a lot of expenses involved: you will need to pay for legal services both in your home country and in the country you are adopting from. There will be expenses linked to the translation of documents, the provision of a 'home study' report on yourselves by a qualified social worker, the maintenance of the baby while all the formalities are being completed abroad, medical expenses if applicable, and finally the travel and maintenance costs for both of you to travel to the country concerned.

It is essential that you only adopt through a reputable agency or orphanage. There have been many stories in the press about disreputable 'agencies' in third world countries, who have been linked to the theft of babies from their legitimate parents in order to sell them to desperate childless couples overseas. The information that you will get about the baby's background will nearly always be limited. A very thorough medical report on the baby is very much in your interests. There is always the possibility that some medical condition may only reveal itself as the child grows older.

Inter-country adoption is perfectly legal as long as you observe the adoption laws both in your home country and that of the child's country of origin. The first essential step is therefore to find out the legal requirements of both. Contact the relevant government department — in the UK the Home Office, in the US the Department of Health — as well as your local authority or state department. You will be given information about the precise Entry Clearance documentation you require and which can usually only be obtained once you have completed all the complex procedures in the baby's country of origin. The frustrations involved as all of this proceeds can seem to be never-ending, so be forewarned. You must also be able to show legal documentation from the child's country of origin. Here, you should contact the relevant foreign Embassy or High Commission in your home country for advice.

Finally, when you have safely accompanied your baby back to its adoptive home, you must seek to ensure that the legal documentation you have obtained (whether it is a guardianship, custody or adoption order) is recognized in your home country. Do not assume that it is. If necessary you must take steps to re-adopt your baby through the courts and also inform your local authority of your intention to apply for such an adoption order.

Do not expect to get a great deal of help from your local authority and certainly the adoption agencies on the whole do not officially approve of inter-country adoption. Their stance seems to be that a baby or child is better off in its country of birth, than being 'uprooted' and losing its identity and culture and background. We do not live in a perfect world. It is going to be many decades before many countries are able to give any priority to coping with unwanted, unloved, and institutionalized children. It must be better to be able to offer them love, security and education now, as a member of your family, even if it does mean uprooting them. Just ask the children! But don't be blind to the problems ahead. Although in this country we are already living in a multi-racial society, will you be able to adapt to having a mixed-race family? How well will you cope with racial prejudice and discrimination against your own child? Will you be able to help your adopted child when eventually questions about his or her origins are asked?

It is so important to be aware of all the potential problems before they arise which means facing up to them even before you embark upon trans-racial adoption. Help can be obtained from the various adoption agencies and patient support groups (page 210).

Finally, there is the question, 'Do we tell our child about the adoption?' 'Yes, you must', is the only answer, and the sooner the better. Children are extremely adaptable. They will accept any fact about themselves so long as they have love and security. There are some excellent children's books available along the lines of 'I'm special, I'm adopted'. The worry that parents may have is, that when at the age of 18 the adopted child has the right to see the original birth certificate, the original parents will be sought out. There is no need to feel threatened or worried about what is really only a natural curiosity. If you cannot create permanent bonds between yourselves and your child in 18 years, there is really no future in the relationship anyway.

In a book like this, I cannot hope to cover the many aspects of adoption. For further information on adoption, you should approach your national adoption agencies as well as your local adoption and family placement services.

10

So near and yet so far

It's difficult to say what is worse — to go through life and never succeed in becoming pregnant at all, or to eventually become pregnant, only to miscarry.

To experience a miscarriage can be a waking nightmare. At one moment, there you are, happy and buoyed up with hope, expectation and joy in the new life you are growing. The next moment you are bleeding and in pain, admitted to hospital, examined by a harassed doctor, told that you are losing your baby, given a D & C, and then sent home — all within 24 hours. Is it any wonder that both of you are stunned and almost in a state of shock? Sadly, to the busy, acute gynaecological ward, a miscarriage is so commonplace and the patient turnover is so rapid, that there is hardly time for you to ask any questions and often no counselling is given. Perhaps all that has been said to you (and it's meant to console you) is that 'It's probably a good thing because it's Nature's Way of getting rid of something that's gone wrong.' Some consolation. The result is going to be predictable.

As far as *you personally* are concerned, you have failed, both as a wife in 'letting your partner down', and as a future mother. Feelings of guilt are common; 'I must have done something wrong'; 'I should have rested more'; 'Oh, *why* did we make love the night before?' 'WHY, WHY, WHY did it have to happen to me?'

To lose a longed-for baby at any stage of pregnancy is going to result in grief. True, it is worse to have a stillbirth or to experience a child dying than to simply miscarry, but it's grief nonetheless and it hurts so much. You must both allow yourselves to mourn for what might have been. Your partner can feel the loss as acutely as you, but may feel that it is unmanly to cry, and that it's unfair to you, especially when you need to have his support so much. It is essential to be able to talk to each other and not bottle it in. Talking to other women who have miscarried is also very helpful, particularly if they have since succeeded in having a baby. This is also where Mum comes in. She can be your biggest comforter of all. If you do not talk to anyone or communicate, the grief is closely followed by anger, at yourself, at each other, and at the doctors who didn't explain; 'Surely they could have done *something* to stop me from miscarrying, although I know that it wasn't really their fault'. If you have unanswered questions, write them down and seek medical advice. There will usually be at least two big questions: 'Why did it happen?' and 'Will it happen again?' Your family doctor and community midwife can answer some of your questions for you, but it is sometimes necessary to seek specialist advice before you try and become pregnant once more.

Gradually the grief settles but it can merge into a long-lasting depression with swings of mood for many months.

The society we live in often appears to be rather cruel to you after a miscarriage. Babies come at you from all directions. Every magazine you pick up falls open at the picture of some little tot, TV commercials praise the softness of a particular brand of nappy, and prams and pushchairs aim straight for you whenever you go out shopping. The comments of well-meaning family and friends can be especially hurtful — 'Snap out of it'; 'Better luck next time'; 'Pull yourself together'; 'Life goes on'. Nobody seems to understand.

But don't make the whole event horrible. Never forget that for a while, a little while, together you achieved something incredible. You started a new life! It didn't work out this time, but it would be sad if grief and bitterness completely blotted out the joy you experienced in your baby in those early days. Perhaps in some way, having experienced the despair over a loss like a miscarriage, we learn to feel more for others who are grieving and can more easily open our arms to them.

In many countries there are excellent national support groups that can fill in all the gaps that exist in counselling and advice (page 210). They inform and help through local groups. Women with similar experiences can meet and talk. They explode many of the myths about miscarriage. I commend them to you.

'Why did it happen?'

Let us look at the whole subject of miscarriage more closely. The definition of a miscarriage is the loss of a pregnancy before the 28th week. The medical term for miscarriage is abortion, which includes both spontaneous abortion and termination of pregnancy. To tell a woman who has lost her baby by miscarrying, that she has had 'an abortion', is insensitive in the extreme and can only provoke upset and anger.

A miscarriage is a very common event. If one looks at all pregnancies, perhaps as many as 45 per cent will miscarry! This very high figure will include the so called 'biochemical pregnancies' which have been detected through IVF programmes, where there are hormonal changes indicating an early pregnancy, but which comes to nothing. We just do not know how often an overdue but heavier-than-normal period is really a very early miscarriage. Many women have undoubtedly had miscarriages without even realizing that they were pregnant at all. Of those pregnancies that become established with a positive pregnancy test, between 15-25 per cent will miscarry depending on the stage of the pregnancy. What this means is that the majority of normally fertile women who have succeeded in having two or more children, will at some time also have had a miscarriage.

Most women who miscarry already know that they are pregnant. They are usually overdue with their periods and have all the symptoms of early pregnancy, such as nausea, increased tiredness, breast discomfort, and more frequent passing of urine.

The first sign of a possible miscarriage is bleeding from the vagina. This in itself does not mean that a miscarriage will necessary follow. Many women can have a slight bleed during the early months of a normal pregnancy, especially at the time that they would normally have had a period if they had not been pregnant. If a miscarriage is going to occur, the bleeding will get heavier and be accompanied by cramping abdominal pains rather like period pains which are really contractions of the uterus. These contractions will cause the cervix to open until eventually something other than blood is seen to pass out of the vagina. This may be the entire pregnancy contained in its sac, or just a portion of the placenta.

There are, therefore, several stages in the progression from the first signs and symptoms of a possible miscarriage, to the final loss of the pregnancy.

Threatened miscarriage

There is usually some blood loss alone. The cervix has not dilated. The treatment is bed rest until the blood loss has ceased for 48 hours, followed by gentle mobilization. Ultrasound scanning should show evidence of a continuing pregnancy with the baby's heart movements being clearly visible.

Inevitable miscarriage

The miscarriage process has passed the point of no return. The cervix is found to be dilating, indicating the inevitability of the loss of the pregnancy. An 'evacuation of retained products of conception' (a more complex form of D & C) is the usual treatment, rather than to wait for you to eventually miscarry yourself. The chief reason for taking this step is that a miscarriage can be a life-threatening situation if the complication of haemorrhage should get out of control. There is no reason to delay carrying out the evacuation of the uterus unless there should be evidence of infection being present.

Complete miscarriage

Sometimes during the actual process of miscarriage itself, the uterus expels all of its contents. This usually only happens in the later miscarriages. An ultrasound scan will show that the uterus is completely empty. Therefore, an evacuation of the uterus is unnecessary.

Incomplete miscarriage

Some tissue has been passed with the blood loss, or an examination has revealed that part of the placenta is stuck in the canal of the cervix. It is in this commoner group of miscarriages that heavy bleeding is most likely. An evacuation of the uterus is then a matter of some urgency. If heavy bleeding does occur, you are given an intravenous drip into a vein in your arm so that blood loss can be replaced if necessary. An injection of ergometrine is frequently given and this causes the muscle of the uterus to contract. This contraction of the uterus squeezes down on the blood vessels in its wall and the blood loss is reduced.

'Missed' abortion

This is a pregnancy that has died in the uterus but has failed to be expelled. There is no sign of the normal progressive growth of the uterus when you attend the ante-natal clinic and often the symptoms of pregnancy have disappeared. Ultrasound scanning of the uterus will show signs of the pregnancy but no movements of the baby's heart will be seen. The treatment here is to evacuate the uterus. There is no desperate urgency to do this, as the baby will probably have died at least several days before. As most women do not like the idea of carrying around a dead baby in their uterus, I feel that the operation should be carried out as soon as possible. You do not need to be admitted urgently unless you begin to bleed which will probably mean that you are at last miscarrying.

Septic miscarriage

Any of the above types of miscarriage can become infected. Ideally the infection should be brought under control before embarking upon an evacuation of the uterus. But if there is heavy vaginal bleeding, the need to control blood loss will break all the rules, and an evacuation of the uterus will be carried out under antibiotic cover.

Recurrent or habitual miscarriage

This is the term used when three or more successive pregnancies unfortunately miscarry.

In the majority of cases of miscarriage, no actual cause can be found. This is always an unsatisfactory and frustrating state of affairs. The following section goes through some of the possible causes.

1. Increasing maternal age

There is no doubt that as your age increases, the miscarriage rate also rises. This is one of the factors that so reduces the chances of treatments like IVF succeeding in the 40+ age group.

2. Poor health

It is not really surprising to learn that miscarriages will occur more frequently if your general health is poor.

Dietary factors

These are of importance, especially your vitamin intake. A deficiency of the vitamin folic acid may predispose to miscarriage. This is found in fresh vegetables and fruit, which are items often left out of the diet of those who are poor, run-down and tired.

In stress states, not only is your fertility reduced because of the raised prolactin levels that occur, but there is evidence to link chronic long-term stress to recurrent miscarriages. Research has shown that if women who have a lot of stress in their lives are given sympathetic support and care during the early weeks of pregnancy, recurrent miscarriages are less likely to occur.

High levels of *smoking* and a high *alcohol* intake are well recognized as being factors linked with both infertility and miscarriages. A baby gets a pretty raw deal in the uterus. By the time you have taken most of the oxygen from your blood for your own use, not much is left for the baby. If, on top of that, carbon monoxide from smoking has used up a good part of the baby's oxygen supplies, you are really asking for trouble. Alcohol has been shown to interfere with the normal fertilization process, so an embryo that is faulty at the start will miscarry.

3. General infections

When these occur in pregnancy they are associated with a greater risk of miscarriage. The baby is unable to tolerate for long the very high temperatures that can occur in illnesses such as kidney infection and 'flu. With the exceptions of Rubella and Cytomegalovirus infections, the common infections will not in themselves damage the baby.

4. Structural abnormalities of the uterus

These can certainly lead to recurrent miscarriages.

Submucous fibroids (Chapter seven) can interfere with the implantation of the embryo.

A *uterine septum*, if present, does not have a very good blood supply, so it is not able to provide sufficient sustenance for a pregnancy should the embryo have implanted on the septum itself rather than on the uterine wall.

Cervical damage from a tear, or over-stretching due to an over-zealous D & C or from a termination of pregnancy, can lead to a permanent weakening of the cervix. From the 15th week of pregnancy, the cervix begins to bear the weight of the contents of the uterus. If the cervix is weaker than it should normally be, it will become incompetent and the pregnancy can literally drop out. In a typical case, the membranes around the pregnancy will bulge through the weakened canal of the cervix. If there is any sudden increase in pressure within the abdomen, say from coughing or straining at heavy lifting, these membranes will rupture draining away the amniotic fluid from around the baby. After a relatively short and painless labour, the baby is delivered. Unfortunately, this usually happens at a stage of the pregnancy when the baby is too premature to be able to survive. When there is true cervical incompetence, this type of late miscarriage will tend to recur in every pregnancy unless additional support can be given to the cervix. This can be done either by repairing any tear before the next pregnancy, or by inserting a special stitch which closes the upper internal os opening of the cervix. This 'purse string' stitch is inserted just after the first three months of the pregnancy are safely passed, so that there is no risk of an early miscarriage occurring after the stitch is in position.

5. Developmental problems in the baby

There is no doubt that many pregnancies will end in a miscarriage because of a failure in the baby's development. Perhaps in these cases Nature really does know best and the pregnancy is 'rejected' by the uterus. The curious feature is that many of the abnormalities seen in miscarriage specimens, can also be found in babies that are born alive. Chromosomal abnormalities such as Down's Syndrome and Turner's Syndrome are commonly found by those centres which are able to carry out a chromosome analysis of miscarried material. Fortunately the majority of these chromosomal conditions are 'one off' problems, with no more than a 1 per cent chance of recurring. Very rarely, one of the parents may be found to carry the particular abnormality in their own chromosomes which then increases the chance of the problem recurring. Why some of the babies with these conditions will miscarry early and others go on to term is not understood. Other structural abnormalities such as the neural tube defects like spina bifida, and major heart conditions in the baby can also lead to the pregnancy miscarrying, although these too can continue for the full term of the pregnancy.

6. Immunological problems

The body will reject tissue from an outside source, for example a kidney transplant, unless that 'foreign tissue' is protected from rejection by suppressing the body's immune response system. It's remarkable that every pregnancy is not rejected, because a baby is rather like a transplant, being made up of genetic material from its mother and 'foreign' genetic material from its father. The reason all pregnancies are not rejected is that the mother's tissues are able to recognize the foreign material in a pregnancy as something special that must be protected. As a result, the pregnancy is shielded from rejection by an 'enhancing antibody'. When a pregnancy occurs in a couple who are very similar in their genetic make-up, the mother is unable to recognize the pregnancy as being any different to herself. The enhancing antibodies do not come into play, the pregnancy is not protected from the 'rejecting antibodies' and a miscarriage results.

This will recur in every pregnancy for that particular couple unless the mother's immune system can be taught to recognize her partner's genetic material.

The basic immunological test is a special blood test called the anti-paternal cytotoxic antibody test (APCA) which determines whether or not you are making antibodies to your partner's white blood cells. If you are making these antibodies, then the recurrent miscarriages are not due to any form of 'rejection'. If, on the other hand, you are not making antibodies against your partner's white blood cells, then 'immunization' using specially treated and purified white blood cells from your partner's blood may be recommended. This should then teach your immune system to recognize genetic material from your partner and to not reject a future pregnancy.

A newer alternative approach to immunization involves the use of a special placental membrane extract in a technique known as trophoblast membrane infusion. This, too, essentially teaches the body that pregnancy tissue in general is to be protected.

'Will it happen again?'
There is some reassurance in the fact that the majority of women who miscarry eventually succeed in having a normal pregnancy with a happy outcome. This being the case, your immediate reaction to losing your pregnancy is to want to get pregnant again as quickly as possible. But just slow down for a moment. Take a while to sit back and readjust to what has happened and to *prepare for next time*. To have 3-6 months off between pregnancies is generally regarded as being sound advice. There is evidence to suggest that to become pregnant immediately after a miscarriage does increase the chances of miscarrying again. I would also think that if you did get pregnant again immediately after miscarrying, you would enter that pregnancy in some degree of mild terror and trepidation. If you wait those few months, you will be able to look back at the pregnancy you lost much more calmly. I want you to be able to say 'What happened last time was very sad, but it was one of those things that happen frequently. I now feel ready to try again and I'm looking forward to it!'

The waiting time need not be wasted. There is a great deal to be done. Antenatal care begins too late in many pregnancies. I am a great believer in both of you being as fit and as healthy as possible, to be tingling with health and vitality when you actually conceive. I am very keen on women who have had a pregnancy problem, like miscarriage, to be on pre-conception multivitamin therapy. I advise that you should be on the multivitamin of your choice for at least six weeks before you conceive and to then continue with it (at normal recommended dosage) throughout the pregnancy.

Make sure that nasty things cannot happen. NO WOMAN SHOULD ALLOW HERSELF TO GET PREGNANT UNTIL A BLOOD TEST HAS CONFIRMED THAT SHE IS IMMUNE TO RUBELLA. DON'T rely on a history of vaccination at school, because at least 5 per cent of vaccines fail to give immunity. Have a blood test!

If you are overweight, slim! You will feel better, look better, and cope better in pregnancy. Take up some sport that you can enjoy together, like swimming or cycling or even simply walking. Get into shape!

If either of you smoke, STOP! Nobody pretends that it is easy, but nothing worthwhile ever is. Stop together, because it's torture if one of you puffs smoke over the one who is trying to give up. Make your home into a smokeless zone. Throw away all your ashtrays (you won't be prepared to tap ash onto your carpet) and when friends come who want to smoke, tell them to go outside. I hope that you would react violently if you saw someone put a cigarette into your baby's mouth. But if you are a heavy smoker, you yourself are willingly doing the same thing to your own baby 20+ times a day! We know that the babies of smokers tend to be smaller than the babies of non-smokers and the chances of their dying during pregnancy (stillbirth) are also higher. Look upon stopping smoking as a joint investment towards the health and future of your baby. Your motivation to stop couldn't be better!

Alcohol certainly reduces sperm production and increases the proportion of abnormal sperm. It is not unreasonable to assume that the fertilizing capability of a drunken and abnormal sperm will be impaired! Alcohol taken in pregnancy can lead to a lethal condition in the baby known as fetal alcohol intoxication syndrome. Why take any chances?

If there has been some major problem with a previous miscarriage, like cervical incompetence or recurrent miscarriage, there is some definite value in being seen by a specialist *before* you present yourself again in the antenatal clinic. Should surgery be considered for submucous fibroids? Should you be referred for immuno-therapy if you have had recurrent miscarriages?

For many years, I have been a believer in the 'good egg', because I found that the miscarriage rate in over 400 of my clomiphene pregnancies was only 9 per cent as opposed to the 15+ per cent for the general population. I felt that if ovulation could be made to be as near perfect as possible, there would be a greater chance of all going well with the pregnancy. This, in fact, has been borne out by IVF observations, which show that eggs vary in their quality and maturity. For patients who have a history of miscarriages, although they have no problem in getting pregnant themselves, I feel that there is a place for deliberately stimulating ovulation with clomiphene to go for that 'better egg'. There is, however, no guarantee. You can still miscarry. I also support the early weeks of pregnancy with a weekly injection of HCG (human chrononic gonadotrophin) 5,000 units which I continue until the 16th week has been reached.

When you do become pregnant again, most of the guidelines to follow are based upon sound common sense:

- Eat well and sensibly.
- Get sufficient exercise and sleep.
- If your work is very strenuous, consider a change or stop altogether.
- Stop smoking and stop drinking alcohol.
- Avoid intercourse during the week that you would have had a period, i.e. at 8 and 12 weeks. If you find it difficult to abstain at these times, at least reduce the depth of penetration rather than thump the cervix and uterus 20 times a minute!

During the first three months of pregnancy, as a general principle, avoid all medications unless strictly necessary. However, remember that for some conditions like severe uncontrollable vomiting in early pregnancy, the condition itself can lead to more problems for the baby than can medical drug therapy.

As soon as your pregnancy has been confirmed, make sure that you are booked in early for antenatal care. The reassurance of seeing a good scan with an active heart beat will do more for you than anything else.

If there have been chromosomal problems like Down's Syndrome in a previous pregnancy, the question of chromosome screening of the baby by either chorionic villus sampling or amniocentesis will probably have been discussed with you before you even get pregnant again.

The pregnancy after a miscarriage is not always easy on your nerves. It can be full of scares and false alarms for you. Every quite normal ache and twinge can cause terror that the same awful thing is going to happen all over again. Don't be worried that the medical and nursing team looking after you will get fed-up with you. You will find that they will do everything possible to reassure you. In pregnancy, false alarms don't matter, but ignoring them might. NEVER FEEL THAT YOU ARE WASTING OUR TIME.

When finally you have the fulfilment and pure joy of holding your own baby, it may surprise you to find that it does not take away the wistfulness over what might have been for the one you lost earlier.

And even as the years go past, every now and then, you will still wonder . . .

11

Twenty questions

This is a chapter of questions and answers. It is possible that your own specialist will handle a particular problem differently but perfectly correctly. There are always going to be different points of view and a variety of means to reach the same objective.

1. *I need to have a salpingostomy operation. I have been told that there is only an approximately 30 per cent chance of success. Would I be better to opt for IVF?*

If each of your fallopian tubes has formed a hydrosalpinx (blocked at the outer fimbrial end), then to all intents and purposes you are sterile. The fact that you have been offered a salpingostomy operation to open up each blocked tube, implies that your specialist does not feel that they are irretrievably diseased or distorted. You say that there is *only* likely to be a 30 per cent chance of success, but that sounds pretty good when compared to your present zero per cent chance of becoming pregnant. Furthermore, if at least one of your tubes remains open after surgery, you will have approximately six chances each year of becoming pregnant.

With regard to IVF ('test-tube' pregnancy), it is important to get this complex treatment into perspective. Looking at the best results, there is not more than a 20 per cent take-home baby rate per treatment. This means that the majority of IVF treatment cycles will fail.

You do not mention your age. If you are in your late 30s, it may be worthwhile to have your attempt at IVF first, as you are running out of time in which to have some prospect of success with this treatment. For this reason, you cannot afford to delay having IVF for too long. If it works, super! If not, well at least you have had your attempt and your surgical option is still open to you. If, on the other hand, you are only in your late 20s or early 30s, then it may be worthwhile to consider surgery first and keep IVF in reserve.

Remember that there is a small but definitely increased risk (2 per cent) of an ectopic pregnancy after tubal surgery. If you should ever be overdue with a period, inform the clinic straight away. Most clinics will have a facility for carrying out very early pregnancy tests which are extremely accurate. Once your pregnancy has been confirmed, the next important move will be to arrange an ultrasound scan of the uterus. The presence of a pregnancy sac within the uterus will mean that you do not have an ectopic pregnancy. Often the scan will need to be repeated, because it has simply been too early in the pregnancy for anything definite to be seen. Should you notice any lower abdominal pains before a conclusive scan result can be obtained, you will be admitted immediately to hospital, so that an ectopic pregnancy can be excluded. To achieve this, a laparoscopy may be necessary.

However, if you are not pregnant within a year of surgery, your specialist may decide to carry out a 'second look' laparoscopy and repeat the dye test. You will then at least know how things stand.

2.   *After six months of taking danazol for endometriosis, we would like to try for another baby. Will stopping danazol allow the endometriosis to regrow?*

Endometriosis is a very common condition and may be a factor affecting 20 per cent of infertile couples. I am pleased to see that you have already had a baby, although you do not make it clear whether or not you had endometriosis before that pregnancy. If you did, and your endometriosis required treatment with danazol before you were able to conceive, this does not, I'm afraid, guarantee that you will be successful once more. If the endometriosis was only diagnosed after your last pregnancy, it will hopefully not be too severe as that would probably have prevented you from becoming pregnant the first time.

Endometriosis is a most curious condition and does not seem to follow any rules. Some patients respond very well to danazol and all signs of endometriosis disappear completely within six months. In others, the deposits of endometriosis can be as large as ever even after a year on treatment. Some women can get pregnant in the presence of endometriosis while others will fail to do so when the endometriosis has apparently cleared up. The best cure for endometriosis is pregnancy itself because during the nine months without a menstrual cycle the endometriosis tissue shrinks away. Yet I have a patient who had severe endometriosis before her pregnancy, not a sign of the condition at her Caesarean Section, and a recurrence of huge chocolate cysts of the ovaries within two years of having her baby.

If you have had six months on danazol, it would certainly be reasonable to stop treatment and give pregnancy a try. I would, however, check with your specialist first in case he has other plans for you. Without a crystal ball, there is no way of predicting how things will go. I think that there is every chance that you will succeed in your wish to have another baby, but there is also a chance that the endometriosis will rear its head again. If within six months of trying to conceive, you fail to do so, your specialist may then recommend a follow-up laparoscopy to reassess the situation.

2. *We have been trying to conceive for six years. Endometriosis was diagnosed. My specialist has offered surgery to remove all affected areas. My main fear is if my tubes are badly infected will they have to be removed?*

I think you are a bit confused here. Endometriosis is not an infection but a common disease process where some of the endometrium lining of the uterus has either been deposited or been developed outside the uterus. The main affected sites are the ovaries, pelvic ligaments and the peritoneum which covers the inner surface of the abdomen. It is interesting that the tubes are nearly always open, even in the most severely affected cases. Remember that the aim of your specialist is to help you to have a baby and not leave you worse off after surgery than before you started. By surgically removing and destroying all visible endometriosis, this can only improve your chances. It is unusual to need to remove a fallopian tube when operating upon endometriosis. There could conceivably be the situation where not only did you have endometriosis, but were also found to have tubes that were thickened and distorted by chronic inflammation. In that case, to leave the tube behind may only increase your chances of having an ectopic pregnancy. If that is indeed the case with you, there is always the extra option of IVF. Please discuss your worries with your specialist before the operation. I am sure that he or she will be reassuring.

4. *I have had two post-coital tests with poor results, so it was recommended that I try douching with bicarbonate of soda. Could you please tell me the 'recipe' for this, also how often to use it?*

The aim of this important test is to confirm that there is no hostility factor between the mucus and sperm and that the sperm are able to survive and remain active for several hours within the mucus. It is also an indirect way of checking on your partner's sperm production.

The test must have been carried out at the correct time of the cycle, namely when you were ovulating. There are a number of situations which will lead to a negative or poor post-coital test:

- If you do not ovulate, the mucus will be thick and glue-like and of such small quantity that it is virtually non-existent, instead of being watery and flowing.
- Your partner's sperm count may be very low (oligospermia) or even absent altogether (azoospermia).
- The sperm must be able to generate enough propulsion to be able to swim vigorously through the mucus and not simply be shaking on the spot.

The idea behind douching with sodium bicarbonate, an alkaline solution, is that it will remove harmful acidity from the vagina and possibly also from the cervical mucus. There is no doubt that the normal healthy vagina is not a friendly place for sperm. Vaginal acidity destroys a good proportion of the sperm that are deposited there. There is also some evidence that douching with sodium bicarbonate will alter the molecular structure of the mucus itself and open up pathways along which the sperm can travel with ease.

The douching should be carried out not less than half an hour and not more than 12 hours before intercourse. So even douching in the evening before you go to sleep will be beneficial if you have intercourse the next morning.

The 'recipe' is as follows: one level teaspoon of sodium bicarbonate powder (also called bicarbonate of soda); (Note: This is NOT the same thing as baking powder. You do not wish to 'rise' or explode!) plus one pint of warm water (a test that it is approximately at body temperature is when you hardly realize that your hand is in water at all).

Mix the two ingredients together. Stir! Now the idea is to get this solution into the vagina. It's not exactly a situation where you can simply say 'open wide' and pour it in! Your clinic or a good chemist shop can provide you with a 'whirling vaginal spray syringe'. The bulb of the syringe is filled up with your warm solution and the nozzle is gently inserted into the vagina. As the bulb is squeezed, its contents are sprayed into the vagina and then trickle out again. The syringe is then refilled and the procedure repeated until the whole pint of solution has been used up. It is best if you are kneeling in the bath while carrying this out so as to avoid flooding!

You will have gathered that I am deliberately making this into a light-hearted event. Otherwise it is very easy for you to regard the douching as something pretty nasty to have to carry out. Remember that intercourse is meant to be fun. If the douching is a bit of a giggle and if your partner laughs at you — spray him (be careful how you hold the douche syringe as the spray comes out sideways and you too could get an eyeful!)

5. *My doctor told me that I have a retroverted womb and he wants me to see a gynaecologist. We have tried to conceive for 18 months with no success. What treatment, if any, can correct this condition?*

A retroverted or backwards tilting uterus is not an abnormal condition and does not in itself cause infertility. On examination the uterus is completely normal and freely moveable both forwards and backwards. Its natural tendency is simply to be tilted backwards because of its shape. This particular shape of the uterus is normal for 15 per cent of all women. The remaining 85 per cent have an anteverted or forwards tilting uterus. It used to be thought that if the cervix was lifted upwards due to the backward tilt of the uterus, semen would only collect in a pool behind it and be unable to enter the cervix. This, I am glad to tell you, is a myth. Semen spreads all over the place in the vagina, absolutely smothering the cervix! The sperm will nip into the cervix like a flash regardless of whether the cervix is pointing forwards, backwards or whatever-which-way!

There are, however, two situations when a retroverted uterus may be associated with infertility: when the uterus is normally retroverted, the ovaries, positioned behind it, tend to lie lower in the pelvis. As a result they may get thumped during intercourse. The ovaries have the same nerve supply as the testicles, and certainly no man would enjoy having his testicles whacked 20 times a minute during a supposedly enjoyable event! Pain on deep penetration at intercourse is going to make you say 'STOP!' and will lead to some reluctance on your part to try again, especially if you know that it will hurt you. Infertility and even a broken marriage can result from your repeatedly saying 'No'.

If pain at deep penetration is causing you to refuse to have intercourse altogether, this state of affairs is going to become intolerable for both of you and cannot be allowed to continue. So what can be done? If when you are examined in the clinic, the doctor finds that pressure on the cervix and ovaries can reproduce the pain you feel at penetration, it is going to be worthwhile to have the uterus drawn forwards into an anteverted position. One old-fashioned but quite effective way of assessing this, is to fit a device into the upper vagina called a Hodge Pessary which tilts the uterus forwards. Although you would be aware of the pessary at intercourse, you should feel no pain. This 'pessary test' would then indicate whether or not it might be worthwhile to hitch the uterus up more permanently. This involves carrying out an operation called a ventrosuspension, where the round ligaments which pass from each side of the uterus to the front wall of the abdomen, are tightened up. As a result the uterus is drawn quite sharply forwards, lifting the ovaries up out of the lower pelvis and 'out of range' during intercourse. The ventrosuspension can either be done as a normal abdominal operation or by means of laparoscopy which can then be carried out at the same time as the dye test to assess the patency of your tubes. While observing through the laparoscope, each round ligament is drawn forwards and stitched to the sheath covering the muscles of the abdominal wall. A word of warning: for a few days after a ventrosuspension you may feel that you will never walk upright again! You will!

In some women, the uterus is actually stuck and fixed into a retroverted position by some disease process. The two main conditions that can cause this are severe chronic pelvic inflammatory disease and endometriosis. In both conditions, there can be dense adhesions tethering the uterus, tubes and ovaries to the back of the pelvis. On examination, the uterus will hardly move at all, totally unlike the normal, healthy retroverted uterus. Pain at intercourse can be a major feature. The retroverted uterus is the result and not the cause of the pelvic inflammation or the endometriosis. A laparoscopy would confirm the situation. The retroverted uterus will now become a part of the whole condition of your pelvis. After discussion, you will need to decide whether or not to have a more major operation, to divide the adhesions, remove or destroy as much visible endometriosis as possible, and even carry out tubal surgery. In the course of the operation, a ventrosuspension would also be carried out, especially if the ovaries were stuck down low in the pelvis and you were complaining of severe pain at intercourse.

I think that it is a good idea to see a gynaecologist, who hopefully will be able to put your mind at rest about your uterus. Possible causes of your mild infertility can also be investigated. Remember that 80 per cent of normally fertile couples will achieve a pregnancy in the first year of trying and the remaining 20 per cent will take two years. So you still have some leeway.

6. *My husband's sperm counts are showing very poor results and it has been suggested that he should consider having a testicular biopsy. If he has this done and a fault is found, will they be able to cure it with drugs, etc.?*

A testicular biopsy is an investigation performed under a general anaesthetic to remove a small portion of the testicle. This is then examined to check on spermatogenesis (sperm production). It is usually carried out when there is confirmed azoospermia (zero sperm count at semen analysis).

If at biopsy, the tissue removed shows normal sperm production, then the azoospermia is due to an obstruction somewhere between the testicle and the outside world. The usual site of obstruction is in the very delicate tubules that pass from the testicle to make up the beginning of the vas. Occasionally microsurgery can be successful, by removing the blocked segments and doing an end-to-end join up.

If, on the other hand, the biopsy shows that the 'factory shop floor' is not producing sperm properly, then the azoospermia is due to a production fault and not to an obstruction.

Unfortunately, the answer is usually of academic interest only, as in most cases, there isn't much that can be done about it anyway. There are only a very few rare causes of azoospermia that can be improved by fertility drugs. The problems is that sperm production is a continuous process, unlike the production of an egg which is a single event in each cycle.

The advice to have a testicular biopsy will most frequently come from a urologist who has developed a special interest in male infertility. Discuss matters fully with your specialist. If your husband's sperm counts are 'in the millions', as opposed to being zero, then options such as intrauterine insemination (IUI) or even IVF may be successful. If his sperm count shows only the occasional sperm, or azoospermia, it is most unlikely that any treatment will have much effect in improving his fertility. In that case, donor insemination and adoption are the two practical options to consider.

7. *My husband has had three sperm counts done, all giving different results ranging from very poor to acceptable. Why is this? (He hasn't taken any medication which might effect the result.)*

If a semen analysis is carried out every week on a completely normal fertile man, the count can quite normally range from 40-200 million sperm per ml. If your husband's sperm counts are at a lower level, he may get counts ranging from a low of 2 million per ml up to a peak of 20 million per ml. This may be why it is taking you longer to conceive. It will only be when his counts are at their highest that there will be a real chance for a pregnancy.

The sperm count will reflect the body's general health in the same way as the condition of skin and hair will. A chronic illness, or even 'flu will affect the sperm count weeks later.

If he has even a moderate intake of alcohol, this should cease. He should stop smoking and also stop having long hot baths if he indulges in this habit. I presume that he has been examined and that the cluster of varicose veins close to the testicle, known as a varicocele, has been excluded.

Do not lose hope. I have known couples where the sperm count has *never* been above 5 million per ml but the quality has been good, and successful pregnancies have eventually resulted. Remember also that artificial insemination using your husband's sperm (either AIH or intrauterine insemination) and IVF are possibilities too.

8. *My husband has a hydrocele. Is surgery the only answer for this?*

A hydrocele is a collection of clear fluid beneath the outer surrounding coat of the testicle. It is thought to be due to an insufficiency of the lymphatic drainage system of the tissue fluids of the testicle. It can be a congenital condition that he has been born with which has only revealed itself in adult life, or it can follow some form of inflammation, infection or injury. They can become quite large and cause discomfort on walking, sitting or attempting to cross the legs. The fluid around the testicle will conserve heat and as a result may affect sperm production.

Even if the hydrocele is not in any way affecting your husband's sperm counts, it is always worthwhile to be referred to a general surgeon or to a urologist. Firstly, your husband will be reassured that the swelling is only a hydrocele, and secondly, the different treatment options can be discussed. If the swelling is insignificant, symptom-free, and not affecting fertility, it may be felt that it is best to do nothing and simply to keep an eye on it. If it is considered best that he part company with his hydrocele, there are two main treatments that can be offered. The first is to draw off the hydrocele fluid under a local anaesthetic. This will relieve the swelling and remove the awkwardness and discomfort it may have been producing. This can do the trick once and for all but sometimes repeated 'tappings' of the fluid are required. If the fluid keeps on reforming and your husband gets fed up at the prospect of constant visits to the hospital to be 'syphoned off', then a surgical approach to permanently correct the hydrocele may be preferable.

9.   *I had two miscarriages at 8 weeks and at 12 weeks before having my baby, now aged five years. Since then we have been trying for another baby, but our only 'success' ended in another 8-week miscarriage last month. Is it possible that the same pattern is going to happen again?*

It's a sad fact that 15-25 per cent of all pregnancies will miscarry. That doesn't make it any easier to bear, even if you do already have a child to hold and love. Recurrent miscarriages are devastating to morale, causing tremendous emotional turmoil and feelings of inadequacy and even guilt. You are probably asking yourself, 'Why should this be happening to me?' With there being such a high overall miscarriage rate, your recurrent miscarriages could be put down to pure chance. The flippant statement 'better luck next time' does hold a gem of truth.

From your history, it certainly does not mean that you are going to lose two pregnancies before every successful one, even though that may appear to be the case. Cling to the fact that you *know* that you can carry a pregnancy successfully. You've already proved that.

For your peace of mind it's worthwhile to make sure that there is no structural abnormality of the uterus that could be causing you to miscarry. Ask your doctor to make an appointment for you to see a gynaecologist. Sometimes the uterus can have a thin central wall or septum. If the embryo implants on this septum instead of onto the normal wall of the uterus, a miscarriage is likely, as the septum does not have a good enough blood supply to nourish the growing baby. The clue to this may come from the D & C operation that is often done after miscarrying, when the surgeon may have commented upon an irregularity in the shape of the cavity of the uterus. A hysterosalpingogram X-ray of the uterus may be recommended.

Pre-conception care is in everybody's interests. Only attempt to become pregnant again when you feel emotionally ready to do so. Make certain that you are both as fit as possible when you do conceive. As soon as you go overdue, get the pregnancy confirmed and book in *early* with your specialist's antenatal clinic. Good luck.

10.   *I have recently read an article on the new treatment called GIFT. I would be grateful if you could tell me if I would be suitable for this. I only have one tube that is patent, the other one was removed following an ectopic pregnancy.*

GIFT (Gamete-Intra-Fallopian-Transfer) is a technique derived from IVF, where the gametes (the sperm and the eggs), are replaced directly into the fallopian tubes. The obvious requirement is that the fallopian tubes are healthy and patent. GIFT is a very logical treatment option to consider in otherwise 'unexplained infertility'.

You have had an ectopic pregnancy and are left with only one tube which you say is patent. Are you just presuming the health and patency of this tube or has this been confirmed by a laparoscopy and dye test *after* you had recovered from the ectopic? I may seem to be nit-picking here, but it is very important. You may have been told that at the time of your ectopic pregnancy operation, the other tube *looked* normal and healthy. From a GIFT point of view, it would not be sufficient to rely upon this observation or even upon a tubal patency test that had been carried out before your ectopic pregnancy.

The fact is, that as you have already had one ectopic pregnancy, you are slightly more likely to have another ectopic in your remaining tube. If you have been told that at laparoscopy, this tube looks perfectly normal and is patent to dye, there is then every reason to hope that another pregnancy will occur naturally without any medical intervention. It may take a little longer than average as you will only be able to get pregnant when you ovulate from the ovary on the side of your remaining tube. This means that you will only have 6–7 chances of conception in a year. If you do become pregnant, it is obviously important to rule out another ectopic pregnancy. This means that if you are late with your period, you must get a pregnancy test done and then get referred urgently back to your specialist. Ultrasound should be able to confirm that the pregnancy is in the uterus. If you are pregnant and experiencing pain in the lower abdomen, it may even be necessary to be admitted as an emergency. A laparoscopy may be required if there is doubt about the site of the pregnancy.

If there was great difficulty in conceiving the ectopic pregnancy, then some form of assisted conception may be worth considering. In view of your ectopic history, I feel sure that most units carrying out this work, would opt for IVF rather than GIFT in order to avoid the chance of a second ectopic pregnancy.

This is something worth discussing with your gynaecologist. You can always be referred to a clinic that can offer both IVF and GIFT where the pros and cons of each procedure will be discussed with you in depth.

11. *Could you please tell me if 'GIFT' would be suitable for someone who has repeated miscarriages (five in all). We have been trying to have a baby for seven years.*

I am afraid that GIFT is not the answer to your problem. You don't seem to have any trouble in actually getting pregnant by natural means. Your problem is to continue a pregnancy regardless of whether it is achieved naturally or by some assisted conception technique.

I can fully appreciate how desperate you must feel. To have one miscarriage is bad enough, but to go through five is to experience a nightmare. Before you attempt to get pregnant again, you *must* first be thoroughly investigated in case there is some correctable factor which is contributing to your recurrent miscarriages. A hysterosalpingogram and a hysteroscopy will show up any septum within the uterus. If you have miscarried five times, a case could certainly be made for surgery to remove any large septum. There is also the whole question of an immunological cause for the failure of pregnancy and whether you may be rejecting genetic material from your partner. You may be suitable for immuno-therapy. You do not mention how far the pregnancies progressed. If any of the miscarriages went past the 15th week when the cervix begins to bear the weight of the pregnancy, this would then suggest the possibility of cervical incompetence. In that case, a supporting stitch around the upper part of the cervix may prevent another pregnancy from miscarrying.

If all tests should be normal, it may be felt that there is a place for IVF but not GIFT. The theoretical advantage of GIFT would be that only 'good quality' eggs and sperm would be transferred into the tubes. However, IVF would have an even greater advantage as only normally developing embryos would be chosen for transfer back into the uterus.

12. *I am nearly 40 years of age and have been trying for a family for 10 years. I didn't have any investigations because I was too embarrassed. Even*

*our family and friends think that we have chosen not to have any children.
Twelve months ago I had to go to my doctor because my periods were
becoming irregular. She has told me that I have a hormone imbalance. We
would dearly love to start trying to conceive again, but feel we may have
left it too late. Can we ask for your advice on this please?*

What a pity that you have delayed for so long before seeking professional advice. It is so sad to find that you have felt too embarrassed
and, I suspect, ashamed to approach anyone until recently.

At the age of 40, your fertility is likely to be reduced and certain
options such as IVF and adoption will not be readily available to you.
Although time is rapidly running out, a pregnancy may still be
possible. However, it is important that you appreciate the obstacles in
your path, and just what it is you may be letting yourself in for.

You will need to be seen speedily by a specialist who will take your
history and then carry out an examination. Initial tests will include
Rubella screening, your pituitary and ovarian hormone profile,
thyroid function tests, and semen analyses on your husband. It may
also be suggested that a laparoscopy and dye test should be carried
out to confirm the normality of your pelvis and also show that the
dye can pass freely through both fallopian tubes. From what you say
about your cycle, I would agree that a hormonal imbalance is likely.
This will then raise the question of fertility drug treatment so that
ovulation will become a regular and predictable event each cycle.
Temperature charts, progesterone assays and even ultrasound may be
used to monitor ovulation. Sperm survival in cervical mucus will be
assessed by the post-coital test. Everything possible should be done
to make you both as fertile as possible.

It may be that in the course of your various tests, some absolute
cause is found for your long infertility history. In that case you will
at least know at an early stage exactly where you stand. If there is a
treatable cause, you will then have an opportunity to become
pregnant, but I strongly feel that you should set yourselves a time
limit, say, your 41st birthday. Otherwise you run the risk of dragging
on with your infertility attempts into your mid-forties! So although it
is stating the obvious, your first trick is to **get** pregnant!

Should you succeed in becoming pregnant, your next trick is to
hang on to it. The miscarriage rate is certainly increased in the older
age group, around the 25 per cent level. There is then the whole
question of screening for Down's Syndrome. At the age of 40 the
chances of your having a baby affected with this condition are about

1 in 80. This means that if you decide not to have a screening test carried out, the odds are still very much in the baby's favour that all will be well. You must remember that the tests themselves carry a definite miscarriage risk of 1 in 150 for amniocentesis and 1 in 50 for chorionic villus sampling (CVS). The whole aim of having such a screening test performed, is, that if a major abnormality is found, the pregnancy is then terminated. Why otherwise put a normal pregnancy to any risk.

Although you may feel 30, I'm afraid that you are not as far as your body is concerned. You are going to find yourself having intensive antenatal care because this will probably be the only pregnancy you will achieve. Full hospital antenatal care in a consultant unit with regular scans to monitor your baby's well-being would be the normal management. Your circulation will not be as resilient as it was even five years ago, so there is a greater chance of your having problems due to a dramatic rise in blood pressure. Admission to hospital for rest, especially nearer the end of the pregnancy is likely. Finally, at the end of the day, there is a much greater chance of you requiring to have an operative delivery by means of a Caesarean Section.

Still interested?

13.   *We have been trying to conceive for 12 months with no success. I am getting worried as my husband wants me to go to see my doctor. Many years ago I had an abortion (my husband knows nothing about this). Will it be in my medical notes? It wasn't done in the area where I now live. Also, if I need to see a gynaecologist, will he be able to tell when he examines me?*

Whatever past medical history you decide to keep secret from your husband is entirely up to you, although you can see now the problems such secrets can seem to cause you. First of all I would *not* recommend telling your husband about the abortion. While it might make you feel better by getting it off your chest, it's not very fair to him, and is, I assume, an event which predates your relationship with him. It is nobody's business but your own.

However, to keep such relevant details from your medical advisors can be most unwise. First of all, there will probably be some mention of it somewhere in your medical records. Remember that these records are confidential and there is only access to them by medical staff. To put your mind at ease, it would be worthwhile to see your doctor at this stage by yourself. Tell him of your worries concerning information of the abortion being accidentally revealed to your husband. I am sure that he will be reassuring and confirm the confidential nature of your records. He will add to your notes a reminder that your husband does not know and is not to know details of the abortion.

Your previous pregnancy history has several implications. Thinking positively, it shows that at that time at least, you were able to ovulate, had at least one patent tube and that a pregnancy could implant itself normally within the uterus. If you were well after the termination, it is unlikely that you developed any pelvic inflammation. Pelvic inflammatory disease causing blocked tubes and subsequent infertility are risks of a termination, although they can also occur in someone without any past medical history at all.

To answer your last question, no, it is not usually possible to tell from a pelvic examination that you have had a previous abortion unless the cervix has been damaged during the operation. But now you are talking of hiding the information from your specialist. If and when you require a referral to hospital, ask your doctor to mention in his letter that you have had a previous termination but that this is a detail not known to your husband and that it is not to be revealed. If your husband is with you when you first attend the specialist clinic, you will not then be asked about any previous pregnancies. It might be best to go to your first clinic appointment on your own so that you can point out to the specialist that details of the termination are not to be revealed to your husband.

Oh, the tangled webs we weave . . .

14.   *I wonder if you can tell me if my fertility has been reduced. Since the birth of my first baby two years ago, my periods have gone from a 26-day cycle to what is now 36 days. Is this normal? We have been trying for another baby for nine months with no success.*

It is not uncommon to find that the cycle changes after having a baby. This is especially true if you were breast-feeding your baby or went onto the Pill. Periods can stop altogether when you are breast-feeding owing to the high levels of prolactin hormone responsible for producing your milk. After stopping the Pill, your ovaries can sometimes take a few months before they decide to work normally again.

If you are now having a 36-day cycle instad of your normal 26-day pattern, this may merely mean that you now have only 10 chances each year of becoming pregnant instead of your usual 14. Your fertility is likely to be completely normal but your fertile phase will be later in the cycle, around day 20-24. Remember that trying for nine months without success does not equal reduced fertility. You have already proved your ability to conceive and have had a super outcome to that pregnancy. Don't lose sight of the time scale — 80 per cent of normally fertile couples will achieve a pregnancy within a year of trying, and the remaining 20 per cent without two years. Unless you are now in your late 30s, I would take no action at this stage other than to keep on trying.

Sometimes a longer cycle can imply that there is a hormone imbalance. If in the next nine months you still don't succeed in becoming pregnant again, a visit to your doctor is in order. A hormone profile will indicate whether there is a possible problem.

15. *After having a laparoscopy I was told that both of my tubes are blocked. It seems to us that our only hope of having a baby is by IVF. How can we find out who will do this for us?*

You seem to have decided that blocked tubes equals IVF. What does your specialist say? If you have been told that IVF is your only chance of conception, I would have to assume that your tubes are too badly damaged for surgery to have a place. You are not in fact actually saying that. If the tubes are not grossly damaged, surgery can offer success rates at least as good as IVF. It is certainly worth your while to look at all the options that may be open to you.

If it becomes apparent that really only IVF can offer you any chance of success, you need then to be referred to an appropriate clinic. Non-private IVF clinics are a rarity, even within the NHS. The capital expenditure involved in setting up such a clinic is considerable, both with regard to the cost of equipment, and personnel. Those units that can offer NHS IVF have horribly long queues, often of several years before a first consultation. Once preliminary tests have been completed, treatment may only be offered after another delay of a year or two. If you are in your late 30s when you are thinking of applying to one of these clinics, don't bother. The delay involved is going to 'age' you past the acceptance level.

The alternative is to use the facilities provided by the private sector. Your specialist will be able to advise you as to where your nearest local private clinic is situated and give you some idea of the costs involved. These costs per treatment cycle may vary considerably and will not include the costs of the drug treatment. It does not follow that the most expensive unit is always the best. No one pretends that the cost is not inconsiderable. It is, but it is also a realistic sum that most couples could save towards, especially if one takes into account the amount of money that may be spent on cigarettes or even on a very modest holiday. If neither your specialist nor your doctor seem able to advise you on where to go for IVF, the patient support groups and other organizations can give you this information.

16. *It has been suggested that we try AID. We wonder if you can tell us who the donors are and also would we be able to meet them?*

Donor insemination clinics will recruit their donors from a variety of sources, but the most favoured source is undoubtedly the university medical schools. There are a number of reasons for this. Medical students are usually present in adequate numbers, are of above average intelligence, have a sense of responsibility towards patients and are probably healthy (or should know if they are not!). While it might be ideal to use a donor of proven fertility, even a previously fertile man's fertility can alter, and it is perfectly adequate to rely upon the normality of the semen analysis. The pool of medical students is a constantly changing one, as the student will tend to move on to different departments of the hospital or even different hospitals. It would therefore be quite remarkable if any one donor were to provide sperm for 10 pregnancies which is usually taken as the limit for that donor. This removes the worry of the chance of children from the same donor marrying each other. It has been estimated that if 2,000 children were born each year as a result of donor insemination, and if there were no more than five pregnancies from each donor, an unwitting incestuous marriage would occur only once in every 50-100 years. So the chances of such a worrying possibility occurring are remote in the extreme.

You raise an interesting point when you ask if you can meet the donor selected for you. It is generally acknowledged that anonymity is essential in donor insemination. Say for a moment that you knew that it was going to be your husband's brother who was going to be the donor. On the face of it, it might seem a good idea. After all, he will be your husband's closest blood relative. Even the physical features will be similar. But whose child is it when you know who the donor is and he knows who you are? Doesn't it raise the potential for all sorts of interference in the child's upbringing? Imagine the problems that would arise if you smacked your child for some misdemeanour only to be told by the donor, 'Stop that! That's my child you're hitting!' It would be intolerable. To use a close friend as a donor has the same dangers without even the benefit of the similar physical characteristics. To be able to meet your clinic donor, to perhaps learn who he is, to bump into him in the street when you are with your baby, is not fair to yourself or to him. There can be no doubt that the anonymity rule is best.

17. *My husband had a vasectomy during his first marriage after having two children. We are desperate to have children in our marriage but his doctor says vasectomy can't be reversed. Would we be entitled to have AID or is it only available for the childless?*

Men who are seeking a vasectomy operation should be offered the opportunity of sperm banking, although this service is only available in the private sector. They can then still keep their options open and, for a modest sum, maintain potential fertility for future use should their circumstances, like your husband's, drastically change. In practice, very few actually take up this offer, in contrast to the number who request a reversal operation.

The consent form for a vasectomy operation is signed by both the patient and his partner. It states: 'I have been told that the object of the operation is to make me sterile and incapable of fathering another child. I understand that the effect of the operation may not be reversible.' Note the phrase '**may** not be reversible'. This is not the same as '*cannot* be reversed'. I'm afraid that your doctor is quite wrong if he has told you that vasectomies cannot be reversed.

The operation is carried out under a general anaesthetic, usually by a surgeon or urologist with an interest in male infertility. It is a delicate but relatively simple operation to perform, with an overall subsequent pregnancy rate as high as 50 per cent.

Don't get too excited just yet, because there is one potential problem. If your husband's vasectomy was performed more than seven years ago, there is every likelihood that he has developed antibodies to his sperm. Before contemplating surgery it would be wise to make sure that there are no sperm antibodies present. If he goes ahead with the reversal in the presence of antibodies, the chances of success are minimal, even though anatomically each vas can be made patent again.

If there are sperm antibodies present, I feel that there is little point in contemplating a reversal operation. Donor insemination would be likely to be far more successful. It is not only available for the childless. It is available as a service to any suitable infertile couple who may require it.

18. *My post-coital test was negative. Does this mean that we should give up trying to conceive?*

No, most certainly not! A negative post-coital test (PCT) does *not* mean that you cannot get pregnant. The PCT is a test of sperm survival in your cervical mucus and there can be many reasons for this test to be negative. For example, the test may have been carried out on the wrong day, you may not have ovulated well in that cycle and so produced only a little mucus; your partner's sperm count may also be at fault or there may be some hostility factor present in the mucus which has destroyed the sperm. Although the PCT is very important, it is only one of the general screening tests carried out on an infertile couple, and not too much can be read into it unless it forms part of the whole picture.

If this is the only problem that has been found, then your clinic will probably wish to repeat the test first of all, and if still negative, carry out more detailed examinations. A sperm invasion test of your mucus by your partner's sperm will show whether there is some factor present which may be preventing the sperm from swimming into your mucus. It also gives your specialist an opportunity to check the quality of the sperm sample. This is a very simple test to carry out which involves simply placing sperm in contact with mucus on a glass slide and observing what happens. A cross-over sperm invasion test may be recommended, where, under the microscope (not in you!), known normal donor sperm are put in contact with your mucus and normal donor mucus put in contact with your partner's sperm. Sperm antibody blood tests on both of you will be carried out as well. In this way further clues as to the cause of the negative test may be found.

If there is a problem, it is usually due to an inability of the sperm to generate sufficient power to swim through even favourable mucus. In this case, it may be possible to carry out intra-uterine insemination (IUI) after first treating the sperm to obtain only the 'best movers'. Should the mucus itself be thick and glue-like, the mucus can be improved with fertility drugs or be completely by-passed, either by IUI or even IVF.

So to give up after a failed PCT is to throw in the towel before battle has even been commenced!

19. *My husband was found to have sperm antibodies. He was treated with steroids which did not seem to help. Although my tubes are patent, we were advised to try IVF. We have now had two attempts at IVF but on neither occasion did fertilization occur. We are so desperate to have a baby but we seem to have tried everything.*

I am sorry to hear that you are having so much difficulty. Sperm antibodies are of two main types, those that tend to stick the sperm together (agglutinating antibodies) and those that reduce the ability of the sperm to swim properly (inhibiting antibodies). They can be extraordinarily difficult, if not impossible, to clear. However, there are usually a number of freely moving sperm swimming between the stuck together clumps of sperm. During the sperm preparation for IVF a special 'swim-up' technique is used whereby the sperm are washed and only the best sperm that can swim up through the culture medium are used. You do not say whether or not a good swim-up result was obtained at your two attempts at IVF.

Steroids in the form of prednisolone have been used with varied success to try and dampen down sperm antibodies. Because this treatment is not without its complications, many specialists are wary of giving steroids for any length of time. It may be that a prolonged course for up to three months will be beneficial, on condition that the man is under close review.

You more than most people will be aware of just how trying it is to go through IVF. If you are contemplating having another attempt at treatment, the clinic concerned may be able to split the eggs obtained between your husband's sperm and donor sperm. If your husband's sperm are able to achieve fertilization, then of course, those embroys would be transferred. If only the donor sperm are able to bring about fertilization, then the treatment will not have been wasted and these embryos could be used for transfer instead. The clinic would obviously need to discuss this with you at some length first.

You do also have the option of straightforward donor insemination. It is reasonable to assume that donor sperm will have a normal fertilizing ability and be able to fertilize your eggs. Your clinic will need to counsel you carefully on this matter, but it may be the answer to your problems, although I agree that it is side-stepping the issue.

20.   *Please can you help us? I am 44 years old and my husband is 49.*
We have been married for 14 years and for the last 10 years we have been
trying to conceive but without success. All our investigations have been
normal although it was once thought that I had a blocked tube. I had tubal
surgery at that time and I was told that my tubes were patent afterwards.
I have had four attempts at IVF and one attempt at GIFT. At each IVF
attempt, 2–3 embryos were transferred. My last IVF attempt was three
years ago. Recently, another specialist has suggested that I have my
laparoscopy repeated. I would really like to have the tubal surgery carried
out again to try and make me more fertile.

No matter how hard some couples try, the final prize of a pregnancy
seems to elude them. You have certainly gone much further than most
in order to try and fulfil your hopes and dreams of having your own
child. Let us just sit back and take stock of the entire situation for a
moment.

At the age of 44 I have to start by saying that time has sadly run out
for you in the race to try and get pregnant. If you were being seen today
with 10 years of infertility, having had *no investigation or treatment at
all*, it would be reasonable to check that you were physically well,
assess the sperm count and give advice on the correct timing of
intercourse with ovulation. Although this may sound callous, the
correct treatment would then be to wish you well. Let me explain.

Every action we take has its consequences. Even if you were to
succeed in becoming pregnant, the consequences you would need to
overcome would be the high miscarriage rate, the 1 in 40 chances of
Down's Syndrome, the probable admission for raised blood pressure
and a probable Caesarean Section. You will probably be saying 'Fine,
I don't mind that, I just want to get pregnant'. But you have been trying
and trying so very hard. Essentially you have unexplained infertility
and have tried almost every type of infertility treatment that exists to
overcome this. A time must come when somebody says, 'Enough'.
Ideally it should be you, but you have now had the carrot of another
laparoscopy dangled at you and you are understandably grasping at
every straw. Well, you are asking me for my advice and I am saying,
'Stop, please'. Live a little now for yourself and for your husband. You
have had such a magnificent attempt and your failure to have your
longed-for baby has not been for the want of trying. There are bound
to be regrets, but the love that you feel that you are bursting to give
to a baby can be channelled in so many other directions.

I do most sincerely wish you well.

12

Looking to the future

The last decade has seen an explosion in the management of infertility. The establishment of in-vitro fertilization has led to the development of a whole range of allied techniques and treatments and also awakened public and official awareness into the needs of the infertile. In the UK, the Warnock Report has laid down guidelines for these assisted conception techniques, including egg and embryo donation, embryo research, as well as discussion on the legal status of children born as a result of donor insemination and egg or embryo donation. As a result of this report, commercial surrogacy has been made illegal. Other recommendations are still to be implemented. The need for trained infertility counsellors has been recognized and courses to begin to fulfil this need have been set up.

In helping you come to terms with your infertility, the role of patient support groups cannot be overstated. They have obtained media attention and have done much to represent the views of their members. The British Fertility Society represents the majority of infertility specialists in the UK and has played a major role in presenting the facts relating to embryo research to the government. If it had not been for embryo research in the UK in the first place, Steptoe and Edwards would not have been able to pioneer IVF. The supporters of embryo research argue that if carefully controlled and supervised research is carried out upon embryos, there is great potential to relieve human suffering, and that it would in fact be immoral *not* to carry out such research. All pro-researchers agree that there must be full legal statutory controls. Embryo research is an emotive issue and really stems from the issue of when you feel that life begins. Is it at fertilization or only when implantation has occurred?

The arguments against embryo research are based upon the

proposition that the embryo has the same human status as that of a child, that it has the basic human right of life, and any research that is done which leads to its destruction should be regarded as murder.

Between these two groups there are a range of views, some suggesting that the only embryo research that is permissible to carry out is research that will actually benefit the particular embryo and so increase its chance of normal development.

So what of the future? What developments are on the horizon which can affect the management of the infertile?

The most exciting developments will come from egg, sperm and embryo research.

There are three major categories of benefit that it is expected research will bring:

1. To improve the treatment of infertility, especially in the areas of male infertility and embryo implantation. If implantation could be improved, IVF would become much more successful and cost effective and may even become a first line of management for many infertility problems.
2. To gain further knowledge about factors that lead to inherited and congenital disease. If gene or chromosome abnormalities could be detected before embryo replacement in couples at risk of passing on a genetic disease to their children, a defective embryo could be discarded for a healthy one. The technique of embryo biopsy whereby a single cell is removed without damage to the embryo has already been established and will give an opportunity to detect the embryo which has a defective gene.
3. To develop more effective contraceptives. The more that is known about the mechanisms that lead to conception, the more likely it will be that better methods of contraception will be found.

The treatment of male infertility leaves much to be desired. Considerable work has been done to assist weak sperm or the sperm that lacks the ability to penetrate and fertilize the egg. In 1987, the technique of stripping the egg of its outer protective zona pellucida layer was described, thereby removing the barrier to weak sperm that could not otherwise fertilize the egg. In 1988, following this work, a technique called **MIST** was developed in Singapore. This stands for 'Micro-Insemination Sperm Transfer'. Using what is known as a micromanipulator, 5-10 sperm are injected through the zona pellucida to bring the sperm and egg into closer contact. The membrane around the egg can then select the sperm that will bring about fertilization. Already, successes have been reported using MIST. Alternative approaches involve the micro-injection of a single sperm into the egg itself, and the drilling of a hole into the zona thereby allowing for easier access by the sperm. While the news of these exciting developments must bring new hope to men whose sperm counts are too poor even to succeed with IVF, it is important to keep them in their proper perspective. They are likely to have very low success rates and also prove to be very expensive. There is also the worry that these techniques may be giving weak sperm an undesirable advantage. Will the use of possibly inferior sperm lead to an abnormal embryo? There is certainly no evidence of this, however, when IVF or GIFT has been successful in men who have exceedingly low sperm counts. There is still a great deal of research that needs to be carried out before MIST can be offered as a method of treatment.

The future of infertility management is exciting. The 'hit and miss' tactics which are still being used, will soon become an eyebrow-raising historic treatment of the past.

13

Coming to terms with childlessness

As infertility treatments continue to be tried on you without success, there comes a point when you will begin to face the possibility that treatment might not work. Many suppress the slightest thought of this, desperately hoping that the clinic will allow 'just another six months on clomiphene'. The time must come eventually, when you have tried everything that is reasonable, and when either you or your specialist will say 'Enough'. It can be a dreadful day when it comes. You will be screaming inside 'How can I just give up?' For literally years you have both been pursuing the goal of a baby. You've lived around temperature charts, had multiple internal examinations, gone through laparoscopies and even struggled through IVF. And the whole lot has come to nothing.

Being infertile is a true grief state, with a real sense of loss for what might have been. To be deprived of being able to hold your baby is like mourning a death. But it is such a waste to now live in bitterness for the rest of your lives. Because you cannot change your infertility, it becomes a fact that you must learn to live with. It is not defeatist to accept that your lives will be childless, but that does not mean that life is now without any purpose. There are other fulfilments in life and other directions in which you can channel your yearning for a baby, and which can still bring you both happiness. But the regret will never go.

It is essential that you can both accept that your infertility has never been a question of 'fault'. Guilt can be a common emotion for you to experience, but this is pointless. You cannot change the fact of the past termination that may have led to pelvic inflammation, or the vasectomy that could not be successfully reversed. These events are past history. You gain nothing by dwelling on 'if only' thoughts. This is also a time when you will need each other's support and strength badly. Don't be surprised if you find that all interest in making love has gone out of the window. Sure, it used to be great, and even when you went to the clinic there was at least a purpose in it. Just now the whole 'exercise' seems pointless. There is nothing unusual in this reaction, and given time, this aspect of your lives together should return to normal. However, if you feel that there are serious problems arising between both of you, you must seek help. Your doctor is a useful first stop. The patient support groups that I continually refer to can be even better. There you will find others in the same situation, or better still, others who have been there and come through it all.

You can find that it is difficult to relate to friends and family who do have children, and you may even find yourself avoiding contact with them. It's not going to be easy, but life isn't easy either. You will have difficult times when someone close to you announces that she is pregnant, or miscarries, or has a baby. You cannot escape and hide away from pregnant women or other people's children. You will see other 'families' and ache inside.

There is a marvellous book, written by Peter and Diane Houghton, called *Coping with Childlessness*. It gives tremendous support and comfort and is beautifully written.

Some infertile patients can have major psychological problems with deeply suppressed rage and even fury at their lack of success in having a family. A fascinating form of treatment for this is dramatherapy. Dramatherapy is able to help you communicate your emotions. By voicing your problem through drama and responding to dramatic images, if necessary using dolls and puppets, you are encouraged to portray your deepest feelings. The dramatherapist is able to interact with you and improve your communication skills. This may sound bizarre, but it certainly is not. Dramatherapy is recognized as being an extremely effective form of healing.

You cannot forget that you are childless; that would be impossible. But a day does arrive when it is not uppermost in your thoughts, a great day when you will realize that you have won and finally come to terms with your situation.

Useful addresses

British Agencies for Adoption & Fostering (BAAF), 11 Southwark Street, London SE1 1RQ. Tel: 0171-407 8800

British Pregnancy Advisory Service (BPAS), Austy Manor, Wootton Wawen, Solihill, West Midlands B95 6DA. Tel: 05642-3225
BPAS have a number of clinics around the country and offer a variety of services including infertility services.

CHILD, PO Box 154, Hounslow, TW5 0RZ. Tel: 0181-571 4367

The Endometriosis Society, 65 Holmdene Avenue, Herne Hill, London SE24 9LD. Tel: 0171-734 4601

The Family Planning Association, 27 Mortimer Street, London W1N 7RJ. Tel: 0171-636 7886
FPA clinics (the above handles referrals only) offer services on contraception and run infertility and psychosexual counselling clinics.

Foresight: The Association for Pre-conceptual Care, The Old Vicarage, Church Lane, Witley, Godalming, Surrey GU8 5PN. Tel: 0142-879 4500

The Institute of Dramatherapy and Dramatherapy Consultants, 37 Chalk Farm Road, London NW1 8AJ. Tel: 0171-267 9649

Institute for Psychosexual Counselling, 11 Chandos Street, Cavendish Square, London W1M 9DE. Tel: 0171-580 0631

The Miscarriage Association, PO Box 24, Ossett, W. Yorkshire WF5 9XG. Tel: 01924 264579

National Association for the Childless, 318 Summer Lane, Birmingham B19 3RL. Tel: 0121-359 4887

Parent to Parent Information on Adoption Services (PPIAS), Lower Boddington, Daventry, Northamptonshire NN11 6YB. Tel: 01327-60295

USA

Child Welfare League of America, 440 First Street NW, Suite 310, Washington, DC 20001. Tel: 202 638 2952

Holt International Children's Services, PO Box 2880, Eugene, OR 97402. Tel: 503 687 2202

National Committee for Adoption, 1930 17th Street NW, Washington, DC 20009. Tel: 202-328 1200
Represents voluntary agencies; publishes Committee for Adoption Directory of Resources

North American Council for Adoptable Children (NACAC), 1346 Connecticut Avenue NW, Suite 229, Washington, DC 20036.
An umbrella organization which links adoptive parents' groups in Canada and the US

Planned Parenthood Federation of America, 810 Seventh Avenue, New York, NY. Tel: 212-541 7800.

Resolve Inc, PO Box 474, Belmont, MA 2178. Tel: 617-484 2424
A counselling, referral and support agency for infertile couples with support groups in over 40 cities

US Department of Health and Human Services, 200 Independence Avenue SW, Washington, DC 20201. Tel: 202-245 6296

Canada

Canadian Fertility Research Association/Association canadienne de recherche en fertilité, 2065 Alexandre de Seve, Suite 409, Montreal, Québec H2L 2W5. Tel: 514-524 9009

North American Council for Adoptable Children (NACAC), 1346 Connecticut Avenue NW, Suite 229, Washington, DC 20036.
An umbrella organization which links adoptive parents' groups in Canada and the US

Operational Coordination Branch, Ministry of Community & Social Services, 700 Bay Street, Toronto ON M7A 1R9. Tel: 416-965 4363

Serena (SErvice for the REgulation of NAtality) Canada, 151 Holland Avenue, Ottawa, ON K1Y 0Y2. Tel: 613-728 6536

Australia

Adoptive Foster Parents Association Inc, PO Box 1030, Woden, ACT 2614. Tel: 06-254 1191

Concern, PO Box 232, Brindale Centre, Wanniassa, ACT 2903. Tel: 06-291 6415

Concern, PO Box 1347, Parramatta, NSW 2150. Tel: 02-484 3769

Concern, PO Box 125, Vermont, VIC 3133. Tel: 03-703 1179

Concern for the Infertile Couple, PO Box 412, Subiaco, WA 6008. Tel: 09-381 9313

ENCOMPASS, PO Box 32, North Hobart, TAS 7002. Tel: 002-72 5993

Endometriosis Association — Victoria, 37 Andrew Crescent, South Croydon, VIC 3136. Tel: 03-879 1276

Friends of Queensland Fertility Group, PO Box 1271, Brisbane, QLD 4001. Tel: 07-353 2948

HOPE Group (IVF), PO Box 520, Miranda, NSW 2228

Hunter Infertility Group, PO Box 462, Raymond Terrace, NSW 2145

IF Infertility Support Group, PO Box 160, Palmerstone, NT 0831. Tel: 089-32 2421

IF Group (IVF), c/- 13 Chiltern Road, Willoughby, NSW 2068. Tel 02-540 2226, 02-623 1868

Infertility Federation of Australasia, PO Box 426, Erindale Centre, Wanniassa, ACT 2903. Tel: 06-291 6341

IVF Friends, PO Box 482G, Melbourne, VIC 3001. Tel: 03-578 2960

JABS, S.E. QLD IVF Support Group, PO Box 6210, Upper Mt Gravatt, QLD 4122

Jigsaw (Association for adoptees, natural parents and adoptive parents), 39 Mainfold Road, Blackett, NSW 2770. Tel: 02-628 8638

Oasis, PO Box 2420, Adelaide, SA 5001. Tel: 08-278 7700

PIVOT Auxillary c/- Reproduction Biology Unit, Royal Women's Hospital, 132 Grattan Street, Carlton, VIC 3053. Tel: 03-439 1928

WISH Group (IVF), PO Box 31, Westmead, NSW 2145

New Zealand

Auckland Infertility Society, PO Box 68-428, Auckland

Christchurch Infertility Society, PO Box 29-188, Christchurch

Department of Social Welfare (adoption advisory agency), Private Bag 21, Postal Centre, Wellington. Tel: 4-727 666

Dunedin Infertility Group, 60 Queens Street, Dunedin

Hawkes Bay Fertility Support Group, 15 Sealy Road, Napier. Tel: 070 35 8975

New Zealand Infertility Society, PO Box 16-108, Wellington

Wellington Infertility Society, PO Box 20-011, Wellington

Glossary of terms

Abortion	The loss of a pregnancy before the 28th week
AIH	Artificial Insemination by Husband (or partner)
Amenorrhoea	Absence of periods
Ampulla	The slightly wider outer end of the fallopian tube closest to the ovary
Anovulatory	Absence of ovulation
Azoospermia	Absence of sperm in the semen
BBT	Basal Body Temperature (the temperature reading at the beginning of the day before any physical activity)
Bicornuate	'Two-horned' developmental abnormality of the uterus
Biphasic	The typical two-level BBT chart where the temperature rise is suggestive of ovulation
Blastocyst	The stage of development of the fertilized egg just before it is ready to implant in the uterus
Bromocriptine	A fertility drug which reduces high levels of the hormone prolactin which may be causing infertility
Buserilin	A drug used to suppress or 'down regulate' the pituitary gland and prevent the release of FSH and LH

Candida

A yeast-like organism ('thrush') which causes a thick white vaginal discharge and itching

Capacitation

The chemical changes that occur in the sperm which enable it to fertilize the egg

Cervical polyp

An overgrowth of the lining of the canal of the cervix to form a fleshy protruberance on a stalk which can bleed

Cervical polypectomy

The removal of a cervical polyp by twisting it off at the stalk

Cervix

The lower opening of the uterus projecting into the vagina

Chlamydia

An organism transmitted by intercourse which in the male may reduce the quality of the sperm and in the female lead to severe pelvic inflammation which can damage the fallopian tubes

Clomiphene

A fertility drug that stimulates the hypothalamus and pituitary gland in the brain to produce FSH and so in turn stimulate production of a mature egg by the ovary

Cold water treatment

A method of reducing the temperature around the testicles to stimulate sperm production

Corpus luteum

The change that occurs in the follicle after ovulation which then produces progesterone

Cross-over sperm invasion test

A test to assess both the ability of a patient's sperm to penetrate known normal cervical mucus and of known normal sperm to penetrate his partner's mucus

Cryocautery

A method of cautery carried out by freezing

Cyclofenil

A fertility drug which may improve the quality of ovulation and the cervical mucus

D & C	Dilatation and curettage — an operation to stretch the canal of the cervix and then explore the cavity of the uterus to obtain a sample of the lining endometrium
Danazol	A fertility drug used in the treatment of endometriosis
Down regulation	The use of drugs to suppress and 'switch off' the pituitary gland so that it does not release FSH and LH
Ectopic pregnancy	A pregnancy that has implanted outside the uterus, most commonly in the fallopian tube and rarely within the ovary and cavity of the abdomen
Ectopy	The reddened 'eroded' appearance of the cervix due to changes in the type of cells covering its surface
Embryo	The early stages in the development of a baby within the uterus before the 6th week
Endometriosis	A condition where active endometrium is implanted outside the uterus
Endometrium	The lining of the uterus which develops to allow implantation of the blastocyst and is otherwise shed with each period
Epididymo-vasostomy	A micro-surgery operation to remove an obstruction to the normal outflow of sperm from the testicle
Fallopian Tube	Tube passing from each side of the uterus towards the ovary
Fertilization	The penetration of an egg by a sperm
Fibroid	A benign (not malignant) tumour of the muscle of the wall of the uterus
Follicle	Cell structures within the ovary that contain an egg
Follicular Phase	The first half of the menstrual cycle when an egg develops to reach maturity

FSH

Follicle Stimulating Hormone leading to the growth of a mature egg in the woman and the production of sperm in the man

Galactorrhoea

The production of milk when there is no associated pregnancy, often due to an increased output of the hormone prolactin

GIFT

Gamete Intra-Fallopian Transfer, an assisted conception technique which has a place in the treatment of 'unexplained infertility'

GnRH

Gonadotrophin Releasing Hormone (also called LH-RH) which stimulates the pituitary gland to release FSH and LH

Gonadotrophins

A collective name for the hormones FSH and LH

Goserilin

A drug similar to buserilin being particularly useful in the treatment of endometriosis and fibroids

Gynaecology

Literally meaning 'knowledge of women'. It is the medical speciality dealing with disorders in the female reproductive system (including infertility)

HCG

Human Chorionic Gonadotrophin, a hormone produced by the placenta, the detection of which is the basis of pregnancy tests

HMG

Human Menopausal Gonadotrophin, refers to the high levels of FSH and LH produced after the menopause, which when extracted from the urine and purified can be used for the treatment of certain types of infertility

Hormone

A chemical substance produced by a gland which is released into the bloodstream and stimulates other glands and organs to function normally

Hydrocele	An excess of fluid around a testicle often enlarging the scrotum
Hydrosalpinx	A fallopian tube blocked at its outer fimbrial end
Hymen	A thin fold of skin protecting the entrance to the vagina in a virgin
Hyperprolactinaemia	Abnormally high levels of prolactin hormone in the blood associated with galactorrhoea and infertility
Hypothalamus	Area of the brain responsible for the control of the pituitary gland
Hysteroplasty	An operation on the uterus to remove a septum and so restore its structure to normal
Hysterosalpingogram	An X-ray taken of the cavity of the uterus and of the fallopian tubes after injecting a detectable radio-opaque dye through the cervix
Implantation	The embedding of the early embryo into the endometrium of the uterus
Impotence	The inability of a man to produce or maintain an erection of the penis
Isthmus	The narrowest portion of the fallopian tube closest to the uterus
IUCD	Intra-uterine Contraceptive Device, or coil
IUI	Intra-uterine Insemination, an assisted conception technique to place specially 'washed' sperm within the cavity of the uterus
IVF	In-vitro Fertilization or 'test-tube' pregnancy, an assisted conception technique, whereby an egg is fertilized outside the body, and the resulting early embryo transferred into the cavity of the uterus

Laparoscopy

The inspection of the pelvic organs by means of a laparoscope inserted through the abdominal wall

LH

Luteinizing Hormone, produced by the pituitary gland, stimulates ovulation to take place, while in the male it is responsible for the release of testosterone from the testicles and in the production of sperm

LUF

Luteinized unruptured follicle — at the time of ovulation the follicle fails to release the mature egg within it

Luteal Phase

The second half of the menstrual cycle which begins after ovulation and continues until the next period commences

Menopause

The 'change of life' when periods naturally stop as the ovaries run out of eggs

Menstrual Cycle

The cycle of events from the beginning of a period until the next period commences

Menstruation

The period which is the shedding of the endometrium if implantation of a fertilized egg does not occur

MIST

Micro-Insemination Sperm Transfer, an assisted conception technique still under development, whereby a single sperm is injected into the egg, or several sperm are placed around the especially prepared egg in the hope that fertilization will occur

Morula

The fertilized egg which after a few days forms a cluster of cells

Mucus

The fluid produced by the glands of the cervix

Myomectomy

The operation to remove fibroids from the uterus

Oestrogen

The female hormone produced by the follicles in the ovaries

Oligomenorrhoea	Periods that are few and far between
Oligospermia	A very low sub-normal sperm count
Oocyte	An egg or ovum from an ovarian follicle
Oophorolysis	An operation to remove adhesions from around an ovary
Orchidopexy	An operation to bring down an undescended testicle and anchor it in the scrotum
Ovarian failure	A state that exists when the ovaries run out of eggs, e.g. at the menopause
Ovaries	The female reproductive organs that contain the eggs and which produce the female hormones oestrogen and progesterone
Ovulation	The release of a mature egg from an ovarian follicle
PCOD	Polycystic ovarian disease
Pituitary gland	A gland beneath the brain which secretes the hormones controlling ovulation and the menstrual cycle, as well as many other vital processes within the body
Premature ejaculation	Male orgasm occurring before or immediately upon penetration at intercourse.
Premature menopause	When the menopause or 'change of life' occurs unexpectedly in the younger woman
Primary infertility	The failure of an individual or couple to have ever produced a child
Progesterone	The female hormone produced by the corpus luteum after ovulation and which prepares the endometrium to receive a fertilized egg
Progesterone challenge test	A test to determine if a woman with amenorrhoea is making adequate amounts

of oestrogen as shown by a withdrawal bleed following a course of progesterone tablets

Prolactin

A hormone produced by the pituitary gland which is responsible for milk production

Prolactinoma

A benign tumour of the pituitary gland which produces an excessive amount of prolactin

Proliferative Phase

Corresponds to the follicular phase of the menstrual cycle when there is growth of the endometrium before ovulation

Retrograde ejaculation

At male orgasm sperm are ejaculated backwards into the bladder instead of forwards along the urethra

Rubella

German Measles

Salpingolysis

An operation to remove adhesions which are tethering the fallopian tube

Salpingostomy

Operation to open up the blocked fimbrial outer end of the fallopian tube

Secondary infertility

The failure of an individual or couple to produce another child when there has been success in the past

Semen

Male ejaculate at intercourse containing the sperm

Semen analysis

An assessment of the number and quality of the sperm within a semen sample

Seminal vesicles

Two glands which produce some of the secretion contributing to the seminal fluid which carries the sperm within it

Septum

A developmental abnormality whereby a 'wall' wholly or partially divides the length of the cavity of the uterus and occasionally the vagina

Speculum	An instrument used (in this context) to examine the cervix while carrying out a vaginal examination
Sperm	The male 'seed' which fertilizes the egg
Spermatogenesis	The complex process of sperm production
Suture	A stitch used at operation to close an incision
Tamoxifen	A fertility drug very similar in its action to clomiphene
Testicles	Male reproductive organs producing sperm and testosterone
Testosterone	Male sex hormone responsible for producing the secondary sex characteristics
Thyroxine	A hormone produced by the thyroid gland which controls the body's metabolic rate
Trichomonas	A sexually transmitted organism which can produce a profuse vaginal discharge and itching in the female, and a urethral discharge and pain on passing urine in the male
UDOR	Ultrasound Directed Oocyte Recovery, a well established method of removing eggs from the follicles during assisted conception techniques such as IVF and ZIFT either via the bladder, urethra or vagina
Ultrasound scan	A method of using high frequency sound waves to visualize structures under examination on a screen
Urethra	The tube along which urine is passed from the bladder to the outside of the body; in the male, semen is also passed out along the urethra at ejaculation
Urofollitrophin	Pure FSH used as a fertility drug especially in the treatment of PCOD

Uterus	The womb, within which the pregnancy develops and grows
Vagina	The female internal genital organ into which the penis is placed at intercourse so as to deposit semen around the cervix of the uterus
Vaginal dilatation	A procedure to stretch the entrance to the vagina if there is undue discomfort which is preventing intercourse from taking place
Vaginismus	An intense form of vaginal spasm which can make intercourse impossible to carry out
Varicocele	Varicose veins around the vas deferens
Vas deferens	The tube from each testicle transporting the sperm towards the urethra
Vasectomy	Male sterilization where each vas is divided and sealed by tying or diathermy
Vaso-vasostomy	The commonest operation performed to reverse a vasectomy — to rejoin vas to vas
Vulva	The external genital organs of the female
ZIFT	Zygote Intra-Fallopian Transfer, an assisted conception technique whereby embryos resulting from IVF are transferred at laparoscopy into the patent fallopian tubes
Zona pellucida	The layer of cells surrounding the egg
Zygote	A very early embryo

Index

abortion *see* miscarriage 172-82
adoption 166-71
AIDS 146
AIH 139
alcohol 51 128
amenorrhoea 79
  post-Pill related 82, 85, 86
  weight-loss related 82
anovulatory cycle 82
artificial insemination 139
  by husband 139
  by donor 142-49
azoospermia 126, 131

Bartholin's gland (Fig. 1) 22
Basal Body Temperature (BBT) charts, 36-41
bicornuate uterus, (Fig. 22b) 113
blastocyst 29
bromocriptine 94-6
buserilin 103, 117, 123, 153

candida 55
capacitation 28
cervical
  cryocautery 112
  ectopy 112
  incompetence 177
  mucus 27, 28, 59
  polyp 110
  polypectomy 110
cervix (Fig. 2) 23
chlamydia 131, 136
clitoris (Fig. 1) 22
clomiphene 84-94
cold water therapy 133

corpus luteum 23
curettage 111
cyclofenil 92

danazol 123
dermoid cyst 125
dilatation and curettage (D & C) 111
donor insemination (DI, AID) 142-49 198
douching 186
down-regulation 102
dramatherapy 207

ectopic pregnancy 29, 192
egg 28
  retrieval (UDOR) 154-5
  retrieval (laparoscopy) 155, 161
  donation 165
endometrium 27
endometrial biopsy 66-7
endometriosis 122-24, 184, 185
embryo 29
  implantation 29
  transfer 157-8
epididymis (Fig. 3) 24
epididymo-vasostomy 135

fallopian tube (Fig. 2) 23
  ampulla (Fig. 2) 23, 28
  isthmus (Fig. 2) 23, 29
  fimbriae (Fig. 2) 23
  patency tests 69-77
  surgery 117-22
fertilization (Fig. 9) 28
  in-vitro (IVF) 151-59
fibroids 114-17

follicle (Fig. 2) 23
  ultrasound tracking 66
  luteinized unruptured (LUF) 78
Follicle Stimulating Hormone (FSH) 21

Galactorrhoea 94
gas insufflation 72
German Measles *see* Rubella
GIFT (Gamete Intra-Fallopian Transfer) 161-4
gonadotrophin releasing hormone (GnRH) 103-6
goserilin 117, 123

hormone assays 41-3, 61-6
Human Chorionic Gonadotrophin (HCG) 31, 92, 158
  beta HCG 159
Human Menopausal Gonadotrophin (HMG) 96-100
  in assisted conception 153, 160, 161
hydrocele 130, 135, 190
hydrosalpinx 72, 120
hymen, 108
hyperprolactinaemia 66, 83, 94-6
hypothalamus 21, 81-2
  failure 103
hysteroplasty 114
hysterosalpingogram 72-3, 116
hysteroscopy 116

implantation 29

impotence 129, 133
inadequate luteal phase 81,
    87 (case 3)
intercourse 53
    painful 54
    timing 39-41

intra-uterine contraceptive
    device (IUCD) 49
intra-uterine insemination
    (IUI) 141, 160
in-vitro fertilization (IVF)
    149-59, 163-4
isthmus 23

laparoscopy 74-7
luteinizing hormone (LH)
    23
luteinizing hormone
    releasing hormone
    (LHRH) 103-6
LH surge 68
luteinized unruptured
    follicle (LUF) 78

male infertility 126-37
menopause 21
    premature 66, 165
menstrual cycle 21-7
mesterolone 134
micro-insemination-sperm-
    transfer (MIST) 205
miscarriage 172-82
    threatened 174
    inevitable 175
    incomplete 175
    complete 175
    missed 175
    septic 176
    recurrent (habitual) 176
    predisposing factors
        176-79
morula 29
multiple pregnancy risk
    clomiphene 85
    Human Menopausal
        Gonadotrophin &
        urofollitrophin 97, 101
mumps 127
myomectomy 116-7

oestrogen 22
oligomenorrhoea 66, 79-80
oligospermia 126, 139-42

oocyte *see* egg
oophorolysis 120-1
orchidopexy 127, 134-5
ovary 21, 23
ovarian cyst 125
ovarian failure 66, 83
ovulation 23, 26
    confirmation 42, 66
    prediction 68-9
    stimulation 79-107
ovum *see* egg

perineum (Fig. 1) 22
perineoplasty 109
Pill 82
    post-Pill related
        amenorrhoea 82, 85, 86
pituitary gland 21, 25, 82
    failure 81
polycystic ovary disease
    (PCOD) 65, 80
polyp 110
polypectomy 110
post-coital test (PCT)
    59-62, 131, 185, 200
premature ejaculation 129,
    133
premature menopause 66,
    165
progesterone 27, 42, 67
    challenge test 84, 86
    day 21 progesterone assay
        64-5
prolactin 65, 66, 94
prolactinoma 95
prostate gland (Fig. 3) 24

rubella 35-6
retrograde ejaculation 129,
    131, 133
retroverted uterus 187

salpingolysis 120
salpingostomy 120
semen 43
    analysis 43-5, 189-90
    infection 136
seminal vesicle (Fig. 3) 24
sperm 28
    antibodies 127, 131, 136,
        201
    invasion test 62
    cross-over invasion test
        63

wash and swim-up 141,
    152, 160
spermatogenesis 127
    alcohol 51
    smoking 51
split ejaculate 132-3
sterilization reversal 119-20,
    122

tamoxifen 94
testicle (Fig. 3) 24
    biopsy 131, 135, 189
    undescended 130
testosterone 65, 66, 131
thyroxine 65
trichomonas 55
tubal patency tests 69-77
    gas insufflation 72
    hysterosalpingogram 72-3
    laparoscopy and dye
        insufflation 74-7
tubal surgery 117-22
    salpingolysis 120
    salpingostomy 120
    reversal of sterilization
        119-20, 122

ultrasonography 66
ultrasound directed oocyte
    recovery (UDOR) 154-5
unexplained infertility 77,
    160
urethra (Fig. 3) 24
urofollitrophin 100-3
uterus (Fig. 2) 23
    septum 113, 177
    retroverted 187

vagina (Fig. 2) 23
    acidity 27
    dilatation 108
    discharge 55
vaginismus 109
varicocele 130
    ligation 135
vas deferens 24
vasectomy reversal 135, 199
    epidiymo-vasostomy 135
    vaso-vasostomy 135
vasogram 131
ventrosuspension 188

Warnock report 203

zona pellucida 28
zygote intra-fallopian
    transfer (ZIFT) 164-5